EMMAUS PUBLIC LIBRARY
11 EAST MAIN STREET
EMMAUS, PA 18049

A CRUSADE FOR
STROKE PREVENTION

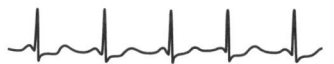

A CRUSADE FOR
STROKE PREVENTION

*A Program for Immediate, Aggressive
Utilization of New Knowledge and Technology
That Could Reduce Strokes by 90 Percent*

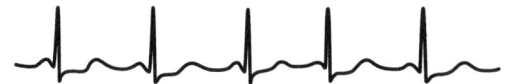

J. CRAYTON PRUITT, M.D., F.A.C.S.
Director of Vascular Institute of Florida

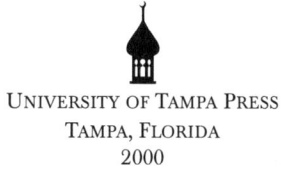

UNIVERSITY OF TAMPA PRESS
TAMPA, FLORIDA
2000

The information contained in this book is not intended to be, nor does it constitute, medical advice. Not every individual exhibits the same symptoms to the same internal or external stimuli, and not every individual reacts in an identical manner to the same medications or treatment. The reader of this book is advised to consult a physician regarding his or her own personal medical condition.

Copyright © 2000 by J. Crayton Pruitt, M.D.
All rights reserved.

Manufactured in the United States of America.
Printed on acid-free paper.∞

The University of Tampa Press
401 West Kennedy Boulevard
Tampa, Florida 33606

ISBN 1-879852-63-2

No part of this book may be reproduced or transmitted in any form or by any means, electronic or mechanical, including photocopying, recording, or by any information storage and retrieval system, without permission in writing from the publisher.

Illustrations on pages 16, 18, 24, and 53 by Laurel C. Lhowe of Medical Graphics, Cambridge, Massachusetts. Medical photographs on the back dust jacket flap and on pages 64 and 65 courtesy of Medical Media Department, Bayfront Medical Center, St. Petersburg, Florida.

Library of Congress Cataloging-in-Publication Data

Pruitt, J. Crayton (John Crayton) , 1931-
   A Crusade for Stroke Prevention : a program for immediate, aggressive utilization of new knowledge and technology that could reduce strokes by 90 percent / J. Crayton Pruitt. -- 1st ed.
     p. cm.
   Includes bibliographical references and index.
   ISBN 1-879852-63-2 (hardcover : alk. paper)iii
   1. Cerebrovascular disease. 2. Cerebrovascular disease--Prevention. I. Title.
RC388.5 .P78 1999
   616.8'1--dc21

                          996775
                            CIP

DEDICATION

*I dedicate this book to my father, J. Major Pruitt, who valiantly
battled the results of two strokes, and to my mother,
Helen G. Pruitt, who loved him enough to keep our family together
and happy in spite of his imperfect condition for
twenty years after his strokes.*

*The book is also dedicated to
Dr. Franklin W. Roush and Ann B. Roush, who
encouraged me to become a physician.*

Contents

Dedication		v
Contents		vii
List of Illustrations		ix
Foreword by William M. Blackshear, Jr., M.D.		xi
Preface		xvii
Acknowledgments		xix

CHAPTER ONE *Understanding Strokes*	An Overview	1
	Father's Stroke	6
	Two Types of Stroke	7
CHAPTER TWO *History, Causes, and Research*	Learning the Causes and Treatments	9
	Recent Studies and Their Findings	12
	The Number One Cause of Strokes: Carotid Stenosis	17
	Risk Factors for Stroke	19
	The Second Most Frequent Cause: Atrial Fibrillation	21
	The Third Largest Cause: Brain Hemorrhage	27
	Attacking the Problem	28

CHAPTER THREE
Prevention of Strokes

	Understanding the Warning Signs	29
	Screening for the Three Major Causes	35
	Making the Final Diagnosis	41

CHAPTER FOUR
Considering Surgery

	Referral to a Surgeon	45
	Knowing the General Procedures	48
	Technique of Carotid Endarterectomy	52

CHAPTER FIVE
Seeking Information

	Key Questions to Ask the Surgeon	67

CHAPTER SIX
Anesthesia

	General Anesthesia	101
	Local-Cervical Block Anesthesia	102
	For Physicians: Preferred Technique for Performing Cervical Block Anesthesia	104

CHAPTER SEVEN
Stroke Prevention Today

	New Emergency Treatment for Acute Strokes	107
	Surviving and Avoiding Stroke	108

	Appendix: An Interview . . .	111
	Notes	125
	Works Cited	131
	Suggestions for Further Reading	136
	Other Useful Resources	137
	Glossary	138
	Index	153

Illustrations

Figure 2.1	Right Carotid Artery and Right Vertebral Artery	16
Figure 2.2	Carotid Stenosis With Small Emboli Breaking off from an Ulcerated Plaque	18
Figure 2.3	A Normal EKG and an Abnormal EKG Showing Irregular Rhythm of Atrial Fibrillation with a Clot in the Atrium	24
Figure 4.1	Acceptable Limits of Mortality and Morbidity for Different Groups of Patients Having Carotid Endarterctomy	49
Figure 4.2	Collateral Circulation to the Brain During Carotid Endarterectomy	53
Figure 4.3	Special Endarterectomy Elevators or Dissectors for Carotid Endarterectomy Procedures	59
Figures 4.4-4.11	Examples of Atherosclerotic Plaque Removed from Carotid Arteries	64
Figure 5.1	Sundt Shunt: Two Sizes	77
Figure 5.2	The Javid Shunt	78
Figure 5.3	The Brener Shunt	78
Figure 5.4	The Pruitt-Inhara Shunt	79
Figure 5.5A	The Inhara-Pruitt Shunt	80
Figure 5.5B	The Inhara-Pruitt Shunt in Position	80
Figure 5.6	The Loftus Shunt	81
Figure 5.7	The Argyle Shunt	82
Figure 5.8	The Pruitt Occlusion Catheter and Pruitt-Inahara Carotid Shunt in Position	84

Foreword

As America ages, the image of the elderly couple living out their remaining years in rocking chairs on the front porch is being transformed into one of energetic, active retirees who want to enjoy the fruits of their lifelong labor to the fullest. Older Americans' greatest fear is not death, but disability. They are most concerned about becoming burdens to their families. There are two main diseases which cripple older Americans and transform them from the active, lively persons they would like to be, into dependents who are forced to rely upon others for care. These disabilities are blindness and stroke. Senior citizens are eager to learn everything possible about prevention and treatment of these two devastating disorders. In this volume, one of America's preeminent carotid artery surgeons, J. Crayton Pruitt, M.D., provides an overview of the causes, diagnosis, and prevention of stroke from the unique perspective of one who has conducted a lifelong "crusade" against this most debilitating illness.

Dr. Pruitt is well-known in medical circles for his expertise in the diagnosis and surgical treatment of carotid artery atherosclerosis, one of the prime causes of stroke in our society.

In addition, he has developed instrumentation which is used worldwide in the operative treatment of carotid artery disease. In this volume, written principally for the layman but useful for the primary care practitioner as well, he provides insight into the intensely personal motivations which spurred his life's work. In the easy conversational style which characterizes his interactions with colleagues and patients and has endeared him to both on a personal and professional level, he provides a step-by-step guide to the causes of stroke, presenting symptoms of the disorder, precise diagnosis of the etiology, and treatment to prevent future strokes.

For many years, clinical research has been infatuated with the prospective randomized study. This is a form of research in which patients are divided into two or more roughly equivalent groups in a random fashion and subjected to two different treatments in order to assess their relative efficacy. It has been touted as the only type of study which provides reliable and definitive data about the efficacy of a particular medical or surgical therapy. Physicians have been cautioned about the pitfalls of relying on "anecdotal" experience–recommendations based on the personal experience of an individual with a limited number of patients. The aphorism "the only thing more dangerous than a doctor with one case is a doctor with two cases" exemplifies this attitude.

Dr. Pruitt has performed more carotid endarterectomies than any other surgeon in the world. Nearly 8,000 patients have benefited from his clinical expertise in this deceptively "simple" operative procedure which demands the utmost of the vascular surgeon's clinical judgment and technical skill. In view of Dr. Pruitt's unique perspective, I believe that there is much to be learned from his "anecdotal" experience. The clinical lessons mastered in the research laboratory of the operative suite based on a vast personal experience should not and must not be overlooked and in many ways cannot be surpassed. The insight he gives patients and physicians into the conduct of carotid endarterectomy, the most common operation for treatment of carotid atherosclerosis, is invaluable. While some of his technical recommendations, such as the use of the "natural thyroid shunt," may not be appropriate for the occasional surgeon, these techniques have worked well for him, and his results are certainly unsurpassed in the literature. Conversely, his insistence on the removal of all diseased tissue by endarterectomy before placing any tacking sutures on a distal intimal edge deserves more emphasis since attempts to "tack down" an edge of residual plaque often result in a technically unsatisfactory end point and lead to postoperative thrombosis.

For the layman who faces the difficult task of selecting a carotid surgeon and understanding the positives and negatives of that surgeon's operative technique for carotid endarterectomy, Dr. Pruitt's compendium of key questions to ask your surgeon will prove invaluable. Similarly, his description of options for conduct of the operation, including anesthesia and cerebral monitoring procedures, is probably the most complete available in the lay literature to date. It is easy to read, and it is written in language which clearly explains the problems, decisions, and reasons to the interested layman.

Undoubtedly, the most controversial section of this book relates to Dr. Pruitt's support for screening large numbers of patients for carotid disease, atrial fibrillation, and hypertension. Devices for the simple measurement of blood pressure in a screening fashion for the detection of hypertension have sprung up in virtually every drugstore in the land, and their routine use is actively encouraged by the best health professionals as well as governmental and private payers. The use of more sophisticated medical screening procedures to detect the other two major causes of stroke—arrhythmias, such as atrial fibrillation, and carotid atherosclerosis—has been much more controversial. Screening evaluation for each of these conditions requires more expensive equipment, and the cost is higher. No insurance plan, private or governmental, reimburses the patient for such screening studies. Furthermore, the specter of exploitation of patients' fears and the potential for over-billing or for performing unnecessary therapy have often been raised with their use. Dr. Pruitt's association with one of the major national screening organizations, Life Line Screening, will subject him to some criticism since he is overtly enthusiastic about this practice. Recent prospective randomized medical series have confirmed the efficacy of carotid endarterectomy for high-grade carotid stenosis in the asymptomatic patient. Patients who are treated in this fashion clearly benefit with a reduced incidence of stroke. Unfortunately, not all patients have warning signs, such as transient ischemic attacks or vertigo, prior to a permanent stroke. One can hardly criticize the concerned layman, particularly if he has evidence of atherosclerosis elsewhere in the lower extremity or coronary arteries, for wanting to know whether he or she is in the high-risk group of patients who has a high-grade carotid stenosis. The nominal cost involved will be well worth the peace of mind to most patients if screening prevents a debilitating stroke which could be fatal or otherwise severely limit his or her ability to enjoy life. Those of us who know Dr. Pruitt also know that his motivation for working with a screening corporation is directly related to his commitment to healing. He acts from an absolute conviction of the efficacy of carotid endarterectomy performed by a well-trained vascular surgeon in the prevention of stroke in asymptomatic patients. His concern for his patients' welfare and his empathy for those who have already suffered the effects of a debilitating cerebrovascular accident are clearly evident in his daily interactions with all of his patients. It is this commendable attitude which has motivated him to encourage stroke screening for older Americans.

Reading this book conjures up the image of a concerned and caring surgeon conducting an intelligent conversation in the office with a patient facing these difficult and daunting decisions. It is the image of a surgeon who believes passionately that treating severe carotid artery atherosclerosis prevents stroke, and that stroke prevention should be one of the utmost priorities of all physicians who deal with older Americans. This book represents a valuable guide for patients and a challenge to physicians to be more aggressive in their efforts at stroke prevention.

As a friend, colleague, and admirer of Dr. Pruitt, I applaud him for his life's work, for his contributions to surgical practice, and for his legacy to patients and physicians as represented in this volume.

William M. Blackshear, Jr. M.D., F.A.C.S.

Preface

As a physician I endeavored to treat a wide variety of surgical conditions, but looking back I was particularly interested, even as a surgical resident, in developing new and better ways to prevent stroke. The fact that my father had a stroke at age fifty-six undoubtedly played an important part in my interest in this field. From the first time I saw the inside of a partially obstructed carotid artery, I knew this was a major problem that was misunderstood by lots of physicians and I was sure the risks of the condition and the early signs and symptoms it sometimes caused were being ignored or not recognized by thousands of patients.

The early papers on the subject written by Dr. Jessie Thompson of Dallas, Dr. H. H. G. Eastcott and Dr. C. G. Rob of London and Dr. Thoralf Sundt of the Mayo Clinic encouraged me to try to learn as much as I could about carotid stenosis which is now known to be the primary cause of stroke.

At that time, the controversy about the significance of carotid stenosis and the proper treatment of the condition was intense, and on several occasions I studied nearly all night to better prepare myself for conferences on the subject that I knew would be attended by neurologists who would debate with me about the relative merits of surgery versus medical management.

Eventually, most of the parameters for medical or surgical treatment were established by large prospective double-blind studies, and the results are discussed in this book along with recommendations for helping to prevent the conditions that predispose to stroke. You will also read how to diagnose strokes if they occur and how to go about getting proper "state of the art" treatment. The treatment options are discussed in detail, including the specific medical vocabulary and correct names of medications, so that you and your physicians will be able to speak the same language. I have tried to explain the unfamiliar terms as they come up, and the new vocabulary should soon become familiar as you read. You will also find a glossary at the end of the book, as well as some illustrations within the text to help clarify the physical problems and the treatment options.

No matter how much time one spends in the study and practice of medicine, the time always seems to be insufficient to the need. There is always more to learn and always more to do. The same may be said, I now see, of writing a book. But just as the good physician must at last turn off the lights and go home, I am at last going to have to let this *Crusade* book go—home to its publisher, and into your hands. Like any crusader, I hope it will be instrumental in achieving victory over stroke.

Acknowledgments

The inspiration, patience, and wisdom of my surgical professors Howard Bradshaw, M.D., Richard T. Myers, M.D., Frank R. Johnston, M.D., and A. Robert Cordell, M.D., is gratefully acknowledged. In addition, the suggestions and ingenuity of Bill McPherson and Toshio Inahara, M.D., in the development of the carotid shunt is acknowledged.

I also acknowledge the help of Rick Morales, P.A., Joyce J. Mendini, R.N., Madeline G. Gallo, R.N., Charlotte A. Womble, Barbara A. Alexander, Sherry L. Imbrior, L.P.N., Joan Klukkert, Karen Grashel, Marcy Winistorfer, Penny Robbins, R.N., and other nurses and office assistants who were knowledgeable, compassionate, and helpful to my patients.

I acknowledge the assistance of Alberto Elizade, M.D., Horst H. Blumberg, M.D., G. Ron Arbisi, M.D., Gordon J. Gilbert, M.D., Eugene W. Hanson, M.D., Juan A. Escobales, M.D., Thomas E. McMicken, M.D., Tomas Y. Paz, M.D., David R. Hirschouer, D.O., Steven R. Cohen, M.D., Garcia J. DeSousa, M.D., William M. Hammesfahr, M.D., Brantley McNeel, M.D., and Harish Patel, M.D., along with approximately eight hundred other physicians who had enough confidence in me and my procedure to refer their patients for surgery on partially obstructed carotid arteries during the controversial period before the national cooperative prospective studies had been completed.

The outstanding performance of many radiologists also contributed valuable insights to this work, and the assistance of Allan E. Katz, M.D., and Chester C. Babat, M.D., is especially appreciated.

I am particularly grateful for the discerning opinions and suggestions about difficult carotid problems offered by my son, Crayton Pruitt, Jr., M.D., F.A.C.S.

I would also like to express my appreciation for the help and patience of Frances Pruitt and my daughters Natalie Judge and Helen Wallace.

Finally, I would like to thank Ellen White, Dr. Richard Mathews, and Ana Montalvo of the University of Tampa Press for their professional expertise in editing and producing this book.

With deep appreciation and thanks to all of you.

CHAPTER ONE

Understanding Strokes

An Overview

A stroke is a sudden neurological change caused by brain damage due to obstruction of an artery or hemorrhage from an artery supplying the brain with blood for oxygen and nutrients.

Remarkable progress has been made in the past forty years concerning the underlying causes of stroke and methods of diagnosing predisposing conditions. Confusion and controversy, however, have caused a lack of focus on the implementation of this knowledge. Stroke is the third largest killer in the United States and the second largest killer in the world. We are still having 730,000 strokes a year in the United States alone at a time when most strokes could be prevented.[1] Fifty million people die in the world each year and about four million three hundred and fifty thousand of these deaths, or 8.7%, are due to strokes.[2]

The exact cause of most strokes was not discovered until late in the twentieth century. Even as late as 1970 it was thought that local thrombosis or clot formation in an artery in the brain was the most common cause. The truth turned out to be that a partial blockage or complete blockage in the carotid artery in the neck is the most common cause of strokes. This condition is secondary to atherosclerosis, which occurs to some extent in all of us, but which becomes excessive in many people. This partially obstructed area often ulcerates which facilitates the formation of a clot in the carotid artery causing sudden obstruction and frequently stroke. In addition, the clots and sometimes particles of calcium can break loose and wash up the neck into a brain artery, causing stroke. That process has now been determined to be the cause of 60 to 65 percent of all strokes.[3] A clot or calcium debris washing up from this area is called an embolus. The underlying condition is called carotid stenosis. In most medical textbooks as late as 1955 carotid stenosis was not even listed as a cause of strokes. Now it is recognized as the most important cause. The reason that pathologists did not discover the true frequency of carotid stenosis and its relationship to stroke seems to be that undertakers use the carotid artery in the embalming process, and therefore the pathologists did not routinely remove the carotid artery for study when autopsies were done. A few pathologists suspected a connection, but it was not until cerebral arteriography was developed that attention was focused on the remarkable degree of obstruction and irregularity in many people who were suffering from stroke. National cooperative prospective studies and international prospective studies were necessary to prove the frequency of the problem.

Various methods were tried to treat the obstructed area in the artery in the neck. Some surgeons preferred to excise the area, some bypassed it with a graft, and others opened the artery, cleaned it out, and sewed it back up. The latter method is called a carotid endarterectomy. This operation has been proven to be superior to medical management without surgery for the prevention of strokes in certain specific groups of patients with significant blockage in their carotid arteries.[4] Though many of the cooperative studies have been completed, some controversy still persists, and it has been a slow process to get all doctors and their patients to accept and use this new information. Eventually these findings should have a dramatic effect on the prevention of stroke.

The second most common cause of stroke is atrial fibrillation, which is an abnormal rhythm in the upper chambers of the heart.[5] Blood tends to form clots in those chambers in this situation, and the clots can often wash up into the brain arteries causing stroke. Atrial fibrillation is estimated to be present in one to two million people in the United States alone, and it causes about 75,000 strokes per year.[6] It is easy, inexpensive and painless to diagnose atrial fibrillation, and treatment with medication can correct the problem or prevent most of the strokes. At the present time fewer than half of those with the condition are on the treatment, even though well-defined treatment guidelines are available.

The third most frequent cause of stroke is hemorrhage into the brain, usually caused by leakage from an artery in the brain because of the effects of hypertension or high blood pressure.[7] It is easy to diagnose those patients with high blood pressure, and excellent treatment is available to lower the pressure after a determination is made about the cause of the hypertension.

All of this boils down to the fact that we now have methods of easily diagnosing the three major causes of stroke and effective treatments are available for all of them. With proper utilization of this new knowledge, we should be able to prevent 90 percent of all strokes *NOW.* This book tells how.

This book is written for the purpose of helping with a more rapid utilization of our new knowledge. A strong position is necessary on the part of those involved in this field to speed up the process for national and global use of the new advances in knowledge and technology. The book will undoubtedly be criticized by some because of the persistent controversy concerning some of its major recommendations. However, these controversial issues should be discussed forthrightly in order that as many people as possible can understand the issues and progress can be made toward winning the crusade for the prevention of strokes.

The information in this book is important and necessary because it reflects an immediate need for using current knowledge to stop the terrible disabilities and large numbers of deaths caused by strokes. The knowledge gained from multiple-prospective, double-blind, national and international cooperative studies has not been widely enough assimilated into day-to-day practice. Many patients and some physicians are confused about what they can do to help prevent this problem. It is a fact that at least one-half of the people who have a stroke have no symptoms prior to the instant that the stroke occurs. Carotid stenosis, a partial blockage in the carotid artery, is the Number One cause of strokes. Many thousands of people have as much as 95 percent obstruction in one or both internal carotid arteries today and are totally asymptomatic. Many of those people will have a stroke in the next few months unless someone diagnoses carotid stenosis and recommends surgical correction by an experienced vascular surgeon, neurosurgeon, or cardiovascular surgeon knowledgeable about the major and minor technical points outlined in this book. This book provides a road map for patients and physicians alike to properly diagnose and treat the underlying conditions which if left untreated will cause a stroke.

Fortunately, ultrasound technology has improved to such an extent that it is easy for well-trained technicians and physicians to screen carotid arteries to determine who is at risk for a stroke due to carotid stenosis. A great many of these patients are totally asymptomatic, and Medicare and insurance companies do not approve of physicians ordering complete, expensive diagnostic studies unless there is an obvious need. However, using the guidelines in this book, if a person spends approximately $35 of his own money for a screening test of the carotid arteries, he can find out if he is one of those people who has a carotid stenosis that is as yet asymptomatic. He will then receive from the screening company a Certified Letter with a report documenting "moderately severe" or "severe" stenosis which he can give to his physician. Armed with this report the physician usually feels comfortable in ordering a complete carotid ultrasound procedure in an accredited noninvasive vascular laboratory, and that test would be covered by the insurance company or Medicare. The complete test is more expensive than the screening test and will cost the insurance company or Medicare approximately $250 to $350. If the complete test confirms the findings of the ultrasound screening, then the physician will proceed with the additional referrals and testing as described in this book.

A similar scenario exists for the strokes caused by atrial fibrillation, which is the Number Two cause of strokes. Screening tests are available as well for prevention of strokes caused by the third leading cause, brain hemorrhage. Medical management, rather than surgery, is usually appropriate treatment for the second and third causes.

Almost all of us have seen friends or family members who have suffered the effects of stroke, and, with an aging population, we are likely to see an increase in stroke. A large number of us would like to have specific guidelines to reduce the chances for stroke in ourselves, our friends, or our family members.

Father's Stroke

One day during my surgical residency I received a call from my mother stating that my father had suffered a stroke and was in the hospital, unable to speak or move his right arm and leg. He was only fifty-six years old at the time and had not had any symptoms prior to the sudden, severe stroke. This event had a huge impact on me and has played an important part in this crusade for prevention of strokes. My father, like thousands of others each year, had an embolus wash from his neck to his left middle cerebral artery, causing a severe stroke. He remained in the hospital for three weeks before being sent home to have physical therapy, occupational therapy, and speech therapy for many months. He never completely recovered, but gradually improved enough that he could talk a little and drive a car. Just two years later he had another stroke. After that, he was unable to talk or even work his zipper. My mother took very good care of him, and he lived a fairly happy life until he died at the age of seventy-three of a heart attack. Today, this type of stroke is preventable.

Classification: Two Types of Stroke

Strokes are classified as ischemic or hemorrhagic.

The ischemic strokes may be embolic or thrombotic. These embolic and thrombotic strokes account for about 80 percent of strokes and hemorrhagic strokes account for about 10 to 15 percent. Auricular fibrillation is responsible for the emboli causing 15 percent of strokes.[8]

Ischemic strokes occur when a cerebral or carotid artery becomes obstructed resulting in a lack of oxygen to the brain tissue. We did not know exactly the high percentage of strokes caused by partial carotid obstruction until 1970. As late as 1955 the Cecil & Loeb *Textbook of Medicine* 9th Edition did not even list carotid stenosis as one of the causes of stroke.[9] Other textbooks of internal medicine did not list it either, because it was unknown. Today, it has been established that carotid artery stenosis in the neck and carotid stenosis with emboli from the neck to the brain cause 60 to 65 percent of all strokes. Most of the clots found on arteriography or autopsy in the middle cerebral artery which were previously thought to be locally formed at the site are now known to be emboli from carotid stenosis in the neck.

All of these can be diagnosed before a stroke occurs and measures can be taken to prevent stroke in each case.

The important thing here is to diagnose the predisposing causes of stroke and take corrective action before the stroke occurs. In the case of carotid stenosis, a screening test using ultrasound technology is inexpensive and accurate for selecting those people who are at risk. In the case of auricular fibrillation, a screening test using an electrocardiogram is inexpensive, readily available, and highly accurate for making the diagnosis that will enable preventative treatment to begin. And in the prevention of hemorrhagic strokes, it is very easy to screen for hypertension by repeated blood pressure checks, enabling treatment for reduction of the blood pressure and thereby reducing the risk of hemorrhagic stroke.

CHAPTER TWO

History, Causes, and Research

Learning the Causes and Treatments

Until 1970, most strokes were thought to be caused by local thrombosis of the middle cerebral artery. A few pathologists, however, had described atherosclerosis leading to partial or complete occlusion in the extracranial segments of the carotid artery and had noted an association with neurological deficits caused by cerebral ischemia. Dr. H. Chiari reported a case in 1905 with atherosclerotic plaque which was ulcerated and expressed the opinion that emboli could break away from the carotid bifurcation and cause strokes.[1] Dr. E. Moniz in Portugal described the technique of cerebral arteriography in 1927.[2] This was an excellent advance in diagnosis that allowed physicians to assess blockage or damage using a simple procedure, and in 1951 Dr. H. C. Johnson and Dr. A. E. Walker reported on 101 cases of thrombosis of the carotid artery diagnosed by arteriography.[3] At about the same time, Dr. Miller Fisher published papers emphasizing the relationship between atherosclerosis of the carotid artery bifurcation and cerebral vascular insufficiency. Fisher published his papers in 1951, 1952, and 1954, and wrote that vascular surgeons might at some future time be able to bypass the area of partial obstruction in the neck to prevent stroke.[4]

The first successful carotid endarterectomy was performed in August 1953 by Dr. Michael DeBakey on a fifty-three-year-old male patient.[5] Preoperatively the patient had suffered a completed stroke. An arteriogram performed postoperatively showed the internal carotid artery to be unobstructed. Prior to the procedure the artery was totally obstructed. The patient survived for nineteen years after surgery and did not have any further strokes, dying of coronary artery disease in 1972. Dr. H. H. G. Eastcott and Dr. C. G. Rob developed an operation for resection of the carotid bifurcation in a patient who had thirty-three transient ischemic attacks and had stenosis of the left carotid bifurcation. An end-to-end anastomosis was carried out following the resection. The patient was completely relieved of symptoms and did not have any further strokes, living to a ripe old age. Eastcott and Rob reported on this case in *Lancet* in 1954.[6]

In spite of these good results, it was felt that strokes caused by carotid stenosis with emboli were probably infrequent, and until around 1970 the major cause of stroke was still considered to be local thrombosis of the middle cerebral artery. In 1970 the results of the first national cooperative prospective study, called the "Joint Study of Extracranial Arterial Occlusion," was released. This early prospective study was carried out in twenty-three major teaching hospitals and reported that carotid stenosis was more common than previously thought. In this study cerebral arteriography was performed for all patients with signs or symptoms of cerebrovascular insufficiency. Surprisingly, 75 percent of the patients in that study were found to have surgically accessible, significant carotid or vertebral stenosis. In the study, carotid endarterectomy was shown to reduce the risk of stroke for certain groups of patients, including those with transient ischemic attacks.[7] For the first time, it was realized that carotid stenosis might be the most common cause of ischemic stroke. Indeed, it has proven to be *the most common cause of all strokes*. It is very important for this point to be emphasized, because technology has improved so that it is easily possible to identify patients with carotid stenosis by using noninvasive methods without risk. Once detected, the areas of obstruction can be removed with minimal risk, so that most strokes can now be prevented by following the simple procedures discussed in this book.

After the preliminary results of the Joint Study of Extracranial Arterial Occlusion were published in 1970, the number of carotid endarterectomies performed in the United States increased rapidly from about 15,000 operations in 1981 to more than 107,000 per year by 1984.[8] These numbers did not include operations done in V.A. Hospitals. Physicians were enthusiastic about the operation, and as a result, a great deal of research concerning cerebral blood flow was carried out. However, some authors reported indications that the surgical complication rate of carotid endarterectomy could be unacceptably high. Dr. J. D. Easton and Dr. D. G. Sherman reported that in Springfield, Illinois, at that time there was a 21.8 percent incidence for acute stroke or death within thirty days of the surgery.[9] In addition, the Newcastle endarterectomy trial which had commenced in 1984 was terminated because of a high morbidity and mortality rate associated with the surgical procedure.[10]

The results of the extracranial/intracranial bypass study were published in 1985, showing an accumulated stroke rate greater in the surgical patients than in the medical patients for those with total occlusion of an internal carotid artery.[11] The initial high morbidity and mortality of the carotid endarterectomy procedure in some hospitals and lack of enough definite evidence that it improved prognosis—in addition to the terrible results obtained in the extracranial/intracranial bypass study—caused the number of patients referred for carotid endarterectomy to gradually diminish. By the year 1990, fewer than 70,000 carotid endarterectomies were performed in the United States.[12] There was a vast difference of opinion between those who were totally convinced that the operation was safe and could be performed with acceptable risks of less than 3 percent for asymptomatic patients and less than 5 percent for symptomatic patients, and other doctors who believed that the operation was of no benefit and perhaps even harmful.

Recent Studies and Their Findings

The controversy continued to get worse and worse, until ultimately the national and international cooperative prospective studies were begun in an effort to solve the controversy. These studies and their findings are as follows:

1. *The North American Symptomatic Carotid Endarterectomy Trial (NASCET)*: Interim results of the study of symptomatic patients were reported on February 21, 1991.[13] The NASCET investigators confirmed that carotid endarterectomy was highly beneficial for patients with recent hemispheric transient ischemic attacks or non-disabling strokes and ipsilateral 70 to 99 percent stenosis. The operation provided a 17 percent absolute risk reduction for this group of patients. In addition, the investigators concluded that there was no benefit from surgery for patients with 0 to 30 percent carotid obstruction.

2. *The European Carotid Surgery Trial (ECST):* This multicenter trial published results in 1991 detailing a beneficial effect of surgery for patients with 70 to 99 percent stenosis who were symptomatic.[14] Patients with 0 to 29 percent stenosis did not benefit from surgery. The conclusions of the ECST were similar to those of the NASCET group. In these prospective studies, the surgical patients received the best surgical treatment available, and the patients treated medically received the best standard medical treatment available.

Nine risk factors for stroke were identified in the NASCET study and the European Carotid Surgery Trial. Those risk factors are:

1. Age greater than eighty years
2. Male gender
3. Systolic blood pressure above 160 mm/Hg
4. Diastolic blood pressure greater than 90 mm/Hg
5. Transient ischemic attacks occurring within the previous 31 days
6. Previous completed stroke
7. Greater than 80 percent carotid stenosis
8. Plaque ulcer
9. History of smoking, myocardial infarction, congestive heart failure, diabetes, hyperlipidemia, intermittent claudication, or high blood pressure.

The odds of having a stroke within two years in the medically treated patients increased with the number of risk factors.

3. *The V.A. Symptomatic Carotid Endarterectomy Trial:* This prospective study demonstrated findings similar to NASCET and ECST. The benefit of surgery appeared to be greatest in patients with internal carotid artery stenosis of more than 70 percent. The results of the V.A. Symptomatic Carotid Endarterectomy Trial were published in 1991.[15]

4. *The Asymptomatic Carotid Atherosclerosis Study (ACAS):* This study of asymptomatic patients with carotid stenosis was begun in 1987 and published its preliminary results on September 29, 1994, following up with detailed results on May 10, 1995.[16] It included patients with 60 to 99 percent stenosis in a carotid artery who were asymptomatic. After publication of the results, the National Institute of Neurological Disease and Stroke released a Clinical Advisory which stated, "Carotid endarterectomy, performed in medical centers with documented combined perioperative morbidity and mortality rates for asymptomatic endarterectomy of less than 3 percent, and on carefully selected patients who continued to have aggressive, modifiable risk factor management is beneficial for patients who meet eligibility criteria for asymptomatic carotid stenosis exceeding 60 percent diameter reduction confirmed by arteriography."[17]

Today 60 to 65 percent of all strokes are thought to be the result of carotid stenosis. It is well-recognized that nearly half of patients who have stroke do not have any prior symptoms.

Ten to 15 percent of cerebral infarctions are hemorrhagic. Many patients who have a transient ischemic attack with complete recovery have a residual infarction demonstrable on CT or MRI brain scans.

It is also true that patients with asymptomatic stenosis sometimes progress without symptoms to total occlusion of an internal carotid artery, which is not usually correctable. The lesion, however, could most often have been corrected if surgery had been performed before total occlusion occurred.

For all of the above reasons, it is extremely important to diagnose carotid stenosis prior to the development of transient ischemic attacks or stroke so that the obstruction can be removed. This could prevent most of the 730,000 strokes that occur in the United States each year.

It is probably wise to recommend carotid endarterectomy for prevention of stroke in those patients who have 60 percent or greater stenosis, whether symptomatic or asymptomatic, if there are no serious medical contraindications. Surgery should only be recommended, however, if the surgeon who is to do the operation has a combined morbidity and mortality for the operation of no more than 3 percent for asymptomatic stenosis, 5 percent for patients with transient ischemic attacks, 7 percent for patients with previous ischemic stroke, 7 percent for patients with recurrent carotid stenosis, and no more than 2 percent mortality for all groups.

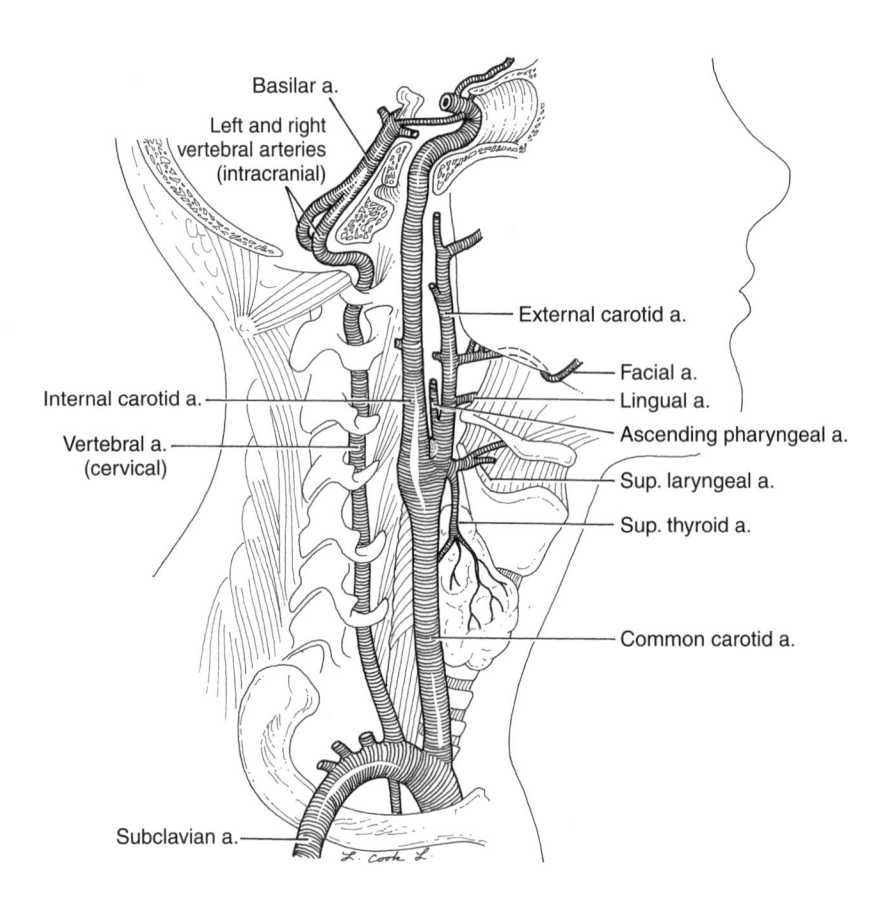

Figure 2.1. Illustration showing right carotid artery and right vertebral artery which carry blood to the brain. There is also a left carotid artery and a left vertebral artery not shown in this picture.

The Number One Cause of Strokes: Carotid Stenosis

The number one cause of strokes is carotid stenosis. The brain receives its blood supply from a left and right carotid artery and a left and right vertebral artery (see figure 2.1). Each carotid artery divides in the middle of the neck into an internal and external carotid artery. The internal artery does not have any branches in the neck. It goes straight to the brain and is the major supplier of oxygen and nutrients to the brain tissue. The external carotid artery has a series of branches which supply blood primarily to the scalp, face, and eye. In the middle of the neck where the carotid artery divides into the external and internal carotid artery, a partial obstruction gradually develops in many people. This blockage is caused by deposits of cholesterol and calcium and is called atherosclerosis or "hardening of the arteries." These deposits begin to form in some men before the age of thirty. Women are usually protected from much of this atherosclerotic process until after menopause. Then women gradually also develop atherosclerosis in this area, often eventually resulting in a significant obstruction. Some plaques are stony hard; others are firm, like tire rubber; and still others are soft and granular. When an obstruction occurs in the carotid area, it is usually asymptomatic until the blockage reaches about 60 percent, at which time ulcerations begin to appear and small blood clots form in the ulcerations. Calcium debris and cholesterol particles can break off along with the small clots and begin to embolize or wash from the neck up into the arteries of the brain. These emboli often lodge in a cerebral artery. The emboli plus the local ob-

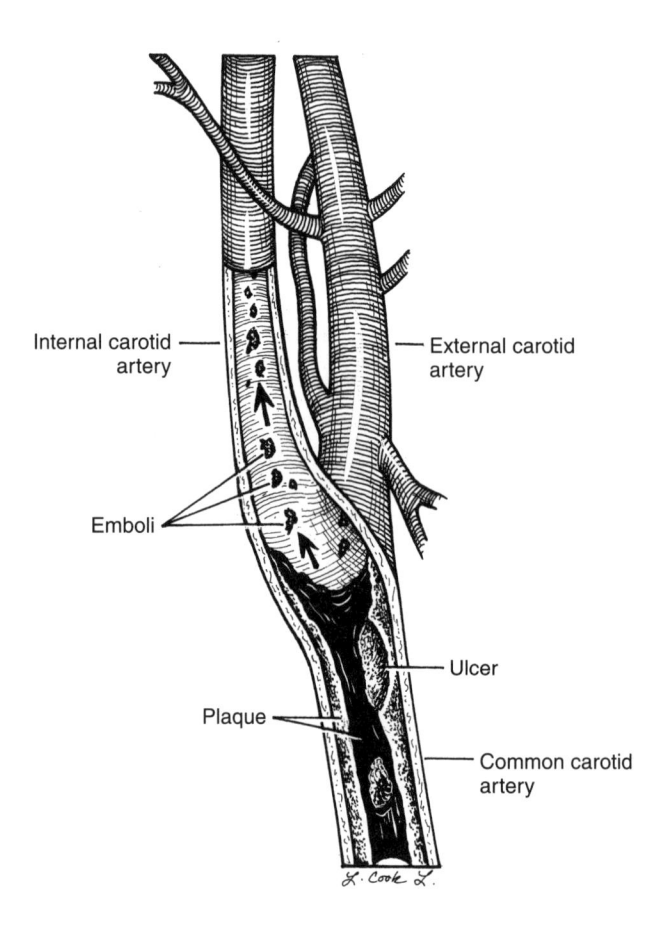

Figure 2.2. Illustration showing carotid stenosis with an ulcerated plaque and small emboli breaking off from the ulcerated plaque. These small emboli can cause transient ischemic attacks. Larger emboli cause permanent strokes.

struction in the neck account for 60 to 65 percent of all strokes (see figure 2.2). Many people have small, transient ischemic attacks (TIAs), which are transient neurologic deficits—brief intervals when normal nerve functions are interrupted. These TIAs include blurring of vision, loss of coordination, slurring of speech, or weakness or numbness in an arm or leg often lasting a few seconds before returning to normal, but sometimes lasting up to twenty-four hours. Those persons who have transient ischemic attacks can be diagnosed and treated to prevent stroke. A surgeon can recommend an operation for removal of the obstructed area to prevent a major stroke from occurring. The problem is that about half of the persons with significant carotid stenosis do not show any symptoms before they have a major stroke. The stroke itself is the first symptom. Therefore, we cannot wait for symptoms to occur before we diagnose and treat.

Risk Factors for Stroke

There are a dozen key risk factors that should be considered when diagnosing and treating stroke:

1. **Family History**—Relatives who have suffered strokes or myocardial infarctions may mean increased risk.

2. **Age**—The risk of stroke advances with advancing age.

3. **Gender**—The male is more likely to develop carotid stenosis but it also occurs in females.

4. **Hypertension**–High blood pressure damages the wall of the arteries and causes an acceleration of the atherosclerosis process.

5. **Previous symptoms**–Transient neurologic deficits occurring within one month indicate unstable or ulcerated plaque, and repeated emboli are common.

6. **Previous stroke**–A prior stroke increases the chance that the problem will recur.

7. **Ulcerated plaque**–Partial obstruction and ulceration in the area of the carotid artery is a significant danger.

8. **Smoking**–Stroke is now one of the well-documented health risks of smoking.

9. **Diabetes Mellitus**–Problems with the body's production or utilization of insulin increase the chances of stroke.

10.. **Myocardial Infarction**–A history of damage to the heart muscle should also be a warning sign for stroke.

11.. **Hyperlipidemia**–Elevation of cholesterol or triglycerides in the blood increases the risk of stroke.

12. **Intermittent claudication**–Pain in the legs when walking due to arterial insufficiency in the legs indicates conditions that may predispose toward stroke.

The Second Most Frequent Cause of Strokes: Atrial Fibrillation

Atrial fibrillation is a condition occurring when the two upper chambers of the heart, called atria, contract in a rapid but irregular and inefficient manner. Physicians call this rhythm an irregular irregularity. The rhythm is not capable of pumping the blood in any meaningful way, so blood remains static in the upper heart chambers long enough to form clots. Some of these clots may break loose from the left atrium and travel through the blood vessels to lodge in arteries of the brain, causing stroke, or they may travel to other organs causing a variety of problems, depending on their ultimate resting place. When one of these clots stops in a cerebral artery, it blocks the blood flow to a portion of the brain, causing an ischemic stroke. More than two million adults in the United States have atrial fibrillation, and the incidence increases with increasing age.[18]

Atrial fibrillation cases can be classified into three different groups or categories:

1. *Valvular atrial fibrillation* – usually secondary to rheumatic fever.

2. *Non-valvular atrial fibrillation* – occurring in association with other significant heart conditions such as hypertension and ischemic heart disease.

3. *Lone atrial fibrillation* – occurring in absence of other significant heart conditions.

In the United States today, the non-valvular type is the most common.

The usual causes of atrial fibrillation include congestive heart failure (in which the heart is unable to pump enough blood to satisfy the metabolic requirements of the body) and coronary artery disease. Atherosclerosis is the most common cause of coronary artery disease. The first symptom of congestive heart failure is usually shortness of breath on exertion. A person will realize that he or she becomes very short of breath when performing activities that formerly caused no problems. The first sign of coronary artery disease is usually a dull chest pain which comes on with exertion or emotional stress. It is called angina pectoris and feels like pressure on the chest.

Structural heart disease is present in 85 to 90 percent of patients with atrial fibrillation. Fifty percent of the patients have hypertension and 25 percent have congestive heart failure. Ten to 15 percent have rheumatic valve disease. Atrial fibrillation affects approximately 4 percent of the population over age sixty and 10 percent of persons over the age of eighty. If atrial fibrillation is diagnosed, the physician should try to discover the cause and, if possible, control the heart rate with medication. He should anticoagulate the patient and consider an attempt to cardiovert with medication or with electrical cardioversion.

Large cooperative trials performed in a prospective manner have definitively demonstrated that long-term anticoagulant use can safely reduce the risk of stroke due to atrial fibrillation for those patients who cannot be cardioverted successfully and monitored in normal sinus rhythm. The anticoagulation treatment helps prevent the formation of blood clots and therefore reduces emobli to the brain. At the present time, however, fewer than half of the appropriate patients with atrial fibrillation are actually on long-term anticoagulation treatment.[19]

The patients with risk factors including hypertension, heart disease, diabetes mellitus, TIAs, or prior stroke have been found to benefit most from the warfarin anticoagulation treatment. If all patients who were proper candidates for long-term anticoagulation were correctly placed on treatment, it is estimated that would prevent more than forty thousand strokes per year in the United States alone.

Atrial fibrillation is fairly easy to diagnose. It can usually be discovered by a screening test with a rhythm strip obtained from an electrocardiograph machine and interpreted by a physician (see figure 2.3). If a problem is detected, the screening company sends a Certified Letter to the patient advising him that the screening test suggests the presence of atrial fibrillation. The patient should take this report to his physician, who should order appropriate further tests to confirm the presence of atrial fibrillation and determine the cause. In most cases, the patient will be placed on anticoagulant medication if no contraindication exists. The patient would then also be referred to a cardiologist who would consider cardioversion, either with medication or with electrocardioversion. If the cardioversion were successful the patient would be placed on medication to help maintain the normal rhythm. If the cardioversion were not successful, the patient would be educated about long-term anticoagulation therapy, and, if agreeable, long-term anticoagulation with warfarin would be instituted.

Atrial fibrillation is primarily diagnosed with a rhythm strip electrocardiogram (EKG). In addition, clots can often be seen within the atria with echocardiograms, which are ultrasound images of the heart obtained noninvasively by an imaging machine using high frequency sound waves. Atrial fibrillation is

24   A Crusade for Stroke Prevention

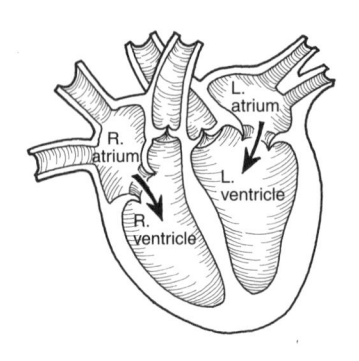

Normal Atrial Contraction

Blood filling the atria from the lungs and body flows into the ventricals with the contraction of the atria.

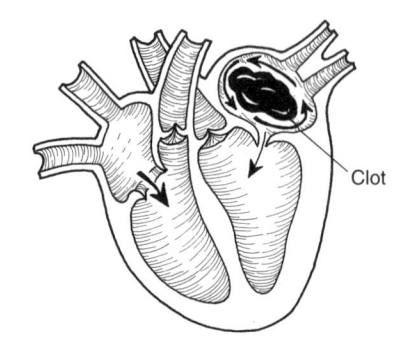

Atrial Fibrillation

Because of the ineffective contractions, blood is stagnant in the atrium where it can clot. The left atrium often becomes enlarged.

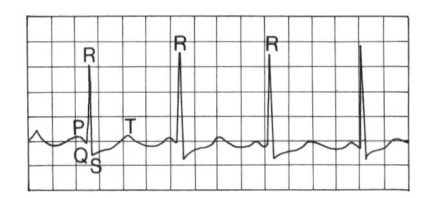

Normal electrocardiogram: The P wave, associated with atrial systole, represents the impulse originating in the sinoatrial node and spread through the atria. The R-R intervals are equal.

Abnormal electrocardiogram—example of atrial fibrillation: This ECG shows baseline fluctuations, indistinct P waves, and varying intervals in the cardiac cycle (The R-R intervals).

Figure 2.3. Cardiac Blood Flow in Atrial Fibrillation

sometimes asymptomatic, but many patients complain of heart palpitations (irregular beating of the heart), skipping of heartbeats, pounding, dizziness, or shortness of breath. The electrocardiogram shows baseline fluctuations and indistinct "P" waves that appear as small ripples of varying size and shape. The ventricular response may be grossly irregular, and R-R intervals may vary significantly.

Once a diagnosis has been made, a physician will frequently prescribe medication to "thin" the blood. Bleeding risks are of concern in patients on anticoagulation therapy, but the large, randomized, prospective clinical trials proved that the increased risk of bleeding was small compared to the large reduction in stroke rate. For every one case of major bleeding in the group receiving the anticoagulant, there were twenty-four cases of stroke in the control group that was not on the anticoagulant.[20]

Those patients who are placed on long-term anticoagulation therapy with warfarin will need to have regular monitoring of their blood coagulation status with the widely used test for assessing the "prothrombin time," or "PT." Historically, the prothrombin time has been measured in seconds, but due to differences in conditions, prothrombin time values are frequently not reproducible from one laboratory to another, sometimes due to differences in the sensitivity of the thromboplastin reagent used in performing the test. As a means of addressing this difficulty, the World Health Organization has introduced use of the International Normalized Ratio (INR), which is a mathematical calculation used to standardize results of coagulation testing. The INR has proven to be reproducible from one laboratory to another, and this measurement is much more reliable than the old "prothrombin time." A proper therapeutic target range for INR values is 2.0 to 3.0. A normal plan to monitor coagulation status would include initial testing every one to three days until the INR is stable, and weekly testing if the INR is unstable. Monthly INR testing to maintain stable INR values is recommended once the target range has been reached. Atrial fibrillation is not the only cause of emboli of cardiac origin, but it does account for 45 percent of them. Other causes include:

a. Acute mycardial infarction with mural thrombus - 15 percent
b. Rheumatic heart disease - 10 percent
c. Prosthetic heart valve - 10 percent
d. Ventricular aneurysm - 10 percent
e. Other - 10 percent

Atrial fibrillation is the most common source of cardiogenic embolism to the brain. Fifteen percent of ischemic strokes are caused by cardiogenic emboli, and 45 percent of cardiogenic emboli are secondary to atrial fibrillation.[21] Atrial fibrillation can be found in about 15 percent of all patients with stroke. About 75,000 strokes per year in the United States are associated with atrial fibrillation.[22]

It is estimated that diagnosing and treating all patients with atrial fibrillation would save at least $600,000,000 in health care costs each year, in addition to preventing more than 40,000 strokes per year.[23]

The Third Largest Cause of Stroke: Brain Hemorrhage

Most hemorrhagic strokes are caused by an intracerebral hemorrhage in which an artery inside the brain ruptures, usually because of hypertension in conjunction with a weakened or damaged blood vessel. As a result of the rupture, blood leaks into the brain tissue causing stroke. This condition accounts for about 10 to 15 percent of all strokes.[24] A second type of hemorrhagic stroke is caused by a hemorrhage occurring between the brain and the skull on the surface of the brain. It usually happens because of rupture of a "berry aneurysm" or "bubble" on the wall of an artery. This accounts for about 10 percent of all strokes. The aneurysms are defects in the artery wall that in some instances can be present from birth. Gradually, these weak spots in the blood vessels balloon out and sometimes leak or rupture causing severe hemorrhage.

A person's blood pressure is considered to be normal if it is 140/90 or below. Keeping the blood pressure within normal limits helps to prevent complications of cerebral aneurysms. Therefore, prompt and effective treatment of hypertension helps to prevent both types of stroke caused by hemorrhage.

In hemorrhagic strokes of either type, the hemorrhage obstructs the flow of blood to some brain tissue causing death of the affected cells. Other parts of the brain tissue are displaced, resulting in neurological changes. Early diagnosis and treatment of hypertension is not too difficult, and it can often prevent these complications.

Attacking the Problem

We can prevent 60 to 65 percent of strokes by correcting carotid stenosis. We can prevent another 10 to 15 percent by diagnosing and treating appropriate patients with atrial fibrillation (half of them are not currently on anticoagulant medication). Finally, we can eliminate another 10 percent by controlling hypertension to prevent strokes caused by cerebral hemorrhage. If we take these three measures, we will have achieved the goal of reducing strokes by 90 percent NOW. Let's get started.

CHAPTER THREE

Prevention of Strokes

Understanding the Warning Signs

Carotid stenosis may be symptomatic or asymptomatic. It may remain asymptomatic even when there is a significant degree of stenosis. This means that a serious condition may exist, even though there are no obvious warning signs. A careful consideration of the causes of stenosis can be revealing.

A condition of stenosis can be caused by fibromuscular hyperplasia or arteritis, but is usually caused by deposits of atherosclerotic material at the carotid bifurcation. This process often begins in men as early as their late twenties and gradually gets worse as they get older. Women are usually protected from the atherosclerotic process until after menopause, at which time they begin to deposit the atherosclerotic material just as the men did earlier. Sometimes, ulcerated plaques will occur when the degree of obstruction is only 50–60 percent. In some of those cases thrombi or particles can embolize from the ulcerated plaques to the brain, causing transient neurologic deficits which last from a few seconds up to twenty-four hours, but no longer than twenty-four hours. If a neurologic deficit persists for more than twenty-four hours, the patient has had a stroke. Sometimes these transient ischemic attacks (TIAs) are recurrent, often occurring many times during the day.

All TIAs should be carefully evaluated. These are **warning signs** for danger for stroke and anyone having a transient ischemic attack should go to the emergency room immediately or call his physician so that appropriate measures may be taken to prevent stroke. Common transient ischemic attacks include:

1. Transient blindness or blurring of vision
2. Transient loss of coordination in an arm, hand, or leg
3. Transient numbness or weakness in an arm or leg
4. Transient slurring of speech
5. Transient expressive aphasia or inability to speak or transit mental confusion
6. Severe, persistent headache
7. Syncope (Fainting)

Each of these attacks has its own characteristics, and it will be helpful to consider them individually in greater detail.

Transient blindness or blurring of vision

A typical patient with this type of attack states that he was feeling normal and carrying out his usual activities when all of a sudden he noticed a blurring of vision, almost like a shade coming down from the top of his left or right eye. This lasted for a few seconds or a few minutes and then the shade lifted itself and the vision returned to normal. The patient may report that he had several of these episodes, all very much alike. Sometimes the event lasts only three to four seconds and the patient does not think that it is significant and does not actually go to the doctor. This type of transient ischemic attack is called "amaurosis fugax." It is characterized by brief episodes of monocular loss of vision which usually comes on suddenly. It may cause a loss of the entire field of vision or a portion of the vision. It is painless, and it may last for a few seconds or a few minutes but never more than twenty-four hours. It is usually caused by embolic obstruction of the ophthalmic artery or a branch of the ophthalmic artery called the central retinal artery which supplies blood to the retina. When the retinal bed becomes ischemic, visual loss occurs. With amaurosis fugax, the emboli break up and the symptoms go away. If the emboli do not break up, partial retinal infarction with permanent loss of vision may result or permanent visual field defects may occur. The eye is truly "a window into the brain," and these small emboli which go to the eye could have gone to the brain instead, causing stroke. Partial obstruction in the carotid artery bifurcation is the most frequent cause of transient retinal ischemia or amaurosis fugax. Transient blindness is an urgent indication for evaluation and treatment. A consultation with an ophthalmologist is frequently necessary to assist with making a definitive diagnosis and to be sure that proper treatment is instituted, not only to prevent strokes but to prevent permanent loss of vision in the affected eye. The ophthalmologist will do a funduscopic examination to look for evidence of diabetic retinopathy, retinal emboli, ischemia, or cholesterol emboli. A type of angiography with fluorescein may be helpful to demonstrate retinal artery or venous thrombosis, and measurements of ocular pressures are necessary to rule out glaucoma. The patient will also need to have a CT scan of the brain or an MRI to help identify stroke. A duplex carotid ultrasound will need to be done to evaluate for carotid stenosis. If the noninvasive testing shows 60 percent or greater carotid stenosis on the side of the embolus, the patient should be advised to have a carotid endarterectomy to prevent additional emboli. The most frequent cause of amaurosis fugax is carotid stenosis, though the emboli can sometimes come from atherosclerotic heart valves or ulcerated plaques in the proximal thoracic aorta. In more than 90 percent of the patients between the ages of fifty and ninety, transient blindness indicates significant carotid artery disease on the same side as the blurring of vision. If the patient goes to a physician, the physician will first take a history concerning the problem and then do a physical examination. As part of the physical examination, an ophthalmoscopic evaluation of the ocular fundi will be performed. This test is critical in the evaluation of carotid circulation ischemia. Retinal emboli may be cholesterol emboli (Hollenhorst plaques), calcific emboli, or platelet emboli. The cholesterol emboli or Hollenhorst plaques are orange-colored material obstructing the retinal vessels where they divide into branches. The Hollenhorst plaques appear larger than the vessel lumen itself. Calcific emboli are white and usually come from calcific valves in the heart; they are frequently found in both eyes. Platelet emboli usually occur due to ulcerated plaques in a carotid artery. They tend to gradually dissolve through a process known as "lysis" and disappear, but sometimes are seen as whitish debris in the vessel lumen.

Prevention of Strokes

Transient loss of coordination in an arm, hand, or leg

A patient who has transient loss of coordination in an arm, hand, or leg will state that he was feeling well until all of a sudden he noticed that he could not hold something with his hand. He continued to drop whatever he was trying to grasp, and he was unable to make his arm or leg do what he wanted it to do. This lasted from a few seconds to a few minutes, and occasionally up to a few hours. If it is a transient ischemic attack, it will completely resolve within twenty-four hours.

The medical diagnosis and treatment of this as well as the other four types of transient symptoms in the following sections are essentially the same. These are discussed in the section below called "Diagnosis and Treatment after TIAs."

Transient numbness or weakness in an arm or leg

A patient with this type of transient ischemic attack has a sudden feeling that an arm or a leg is "asleep," the arm feels heavy, or the leg is not strong enough to hold him up. This type of TIA could last seconds, minutes, or hours, but if it is a transient ischemic attack it will resolve within twenty-four hours.

Transient slurring of speech

A patient with this type of transient ischemic attack will state that the tongue felt thickened and he or she could not pronounce words properly. There is loss of coordination of the tongue itself. He could not say the words clearly that he wanted to say. The problem could last seconds, minutes, or hours, but will completely resolve within twenty-four hours if it is a transient ischemic attack.

Transient expressive aphasia or inability to speak or transit mental confusion

A person with this type of TIA suddenly is unable to express himself. He knows what he wants to say, but the words will not come out. If it is a TIA it will resolve within twenty-four hours.

Severe, persistent headache

Severe, persistent headache can be another type of transient ischemic attack. If it lasts more than twenty-four hours it could mean that a completed stroke has occurred.

Syncope (Fainting)

Severe dizziness or actual syncope is a type of transient ischemic attack which occasionally comes from carotid distribution, but often is caused by partial obstruction due to emboli in the posterior or vertebral circulatory system.

Diagnosis and Treatment after TIAs

If a person has any of the above transient ischemic attacks, he should CALL HIS PHYSICIAN immediately and should proceed straight to the emergency room of a hospital!

Too many people have transient ischemic attacks which are brief and usually painless; the patients ignore the problems and do not seek medical help because the symptoms disappear. It should be emphasized that these transient ischemic attacks are ominous signs and should not be taken lightly. They definitely indicate that the patient is at greatly increased risk of having a stroke within thirty days unless measures are taken to diagnose and treat the underlying cause, which is usually carotid stenosis.

Screening for the Three Major Causes

Screening for Carotid Stenosis

If everyone who were going to have a stroke had a symptom first, then there would not be a problem in diagnosing this condition before the stroke occurred. It is true, however, that at least half of the people who have a stroke do not have any prior transient ischemic attacks. The stroke is the first event. It is, therefore, necessary to perform carotid screening tests to determine which patients are at risk because of significant carotid stenosis but are still asymptomatic. When a patient sees his family physician, a part of the physical examination involves listening to the carotid artery with a stethoscope. In many of these asymptomatic patients the physician hears a noise called a "bruit" with each heartbeat which is a "swishing" sound that is present in many people who have a partial blockage. All of those people should be sent for a carotid ultrasound test to see if there is a significant obstruction. Unfortunately, however, many people with even a very severe carotid stenosis do not have bruits. Therefore, listening with a stethoscope or even a hand-held Doppler device is not adequate. It is necessary to do screening tests to locate those people who are at risk.

At what age should a person begin having ultrasound screening tests to rule out significant asymptomatic carotid stenosis? Consider these facts:

Dorland's Medical Dictionary defines screening as "a mass examination of the population to detect the existence of a particular disease." In the case of screening for carotid stenosis, the best test is an ultrasound test. Although the slightly abbreviated procedure is not a thorough examination of those arteries, it is extensive enough to separate those who have moderately severe or severe stenosis from those who do not have any significant blockage. The test is painless, harmless, and inexpensive.

It is estimated that 650,000 to 730,000 strokes occur in the United States every year. Approximately 60 to 65 percent—or 448,000—of those strokes are due to partial obstruction of the carotid arteries in the neck. The others are caused by one of eighteen other causes, but the majority are caused by emboli from the heart secondary to atrial fibrillation (abnormal rhythm) or hemorrhage into the brain primarily secondary to hypertension. It is possible to screen large groups of people to discover all three of these conditions and choose, on the basis of a positive screening test, which ones need to have further testing to confirm the diagnosis. It is estimated that about one-half of the 420,000 strokes that happen annually due to carotid stenosis occur in asymptomatic people. The Asymptomatic Carotid Atherosclerotic Study (ACAS) proved that carotid endarterectomy, when performed by experienced vascular surgeons, was superior to the best medical management for preventing stroke.[1] Therefore, it is important to screen asymptomatic persons over the age of fifty to discover those who are at risk for a stroke.

If a person, either male or female, is screend and found to have NO atherosclerotic plaques in the carotid arteries, another screening test is not necessary for about three years. If he or she is found to have a MILD amount of atherosclerotic plaque, another test should be done in two years. If a MILD TO MODERATE amount of plaque is reported, another test should be done in one year. And if a MODERATE TO SEVERE amount of plaque or a SEVERE amount of plaque is reported, instructions will be included with the report advising that an appointment be made with his or her personal physician. Usually at that time the physician will suggest ordering a more complete ultrasound test at an accredited vascular laboratory. Whether or not treatment is necessary will depend on the confirmation of significant stenosis by the more complete test. If a person has a family history of strokes at an early age or if there are risk factors involved such as diabetes, hypertension, smoking, or high cholesterol, the first screening test should be done at age forty instead of age fifty. There are several different companies and organizations that provide screening tests for carotid arteries and each of them has slightly different criteria for deciding when to send a report suggesting the need for additional testing.

The National Stroke Association has recommended a program for screening for carotid artery stenosis, atrial fibrillation, and hypertension in all persons over fifty years of age.[2] The stroke screening program sponsored by the National Stroke Association was started in 1993. It was established to encourage local hospitals to encourage stroke prevention screenings. The rationale and goals of the National Stroke Association program were stated to be:

- Reduce the number of strokes by public education and stroke risk screening to detect and manage stroke risk factors.
- Reach at-risk populations such as older adults and African-Americans.
- Increase public awareness of modifiable stroke risk factors.
- Encourage as many people as possible to attend stroke prevention screenings.
- Pay special attention to the detection of untreated hypertension and atrial fibrillation.

- Obtain and evaluate participant screening data.
- Promote individual responsibility for seeking medical follow-up.
- Establish follow-up procedures for at risk individuals.
- Encourage community health care organizations to conduct screenings.

Screening methods for hypertension or atrial fibrillation are similar in most organizations but differ in their approach for screening for carotid stenosis.

Screening methods vary from simply listening to the carotid artery with a stethoscope, listening to the carotid artery with a hand-held Doppler, or performing an abbreviated color flow duplex ultrasound test. The National Stroke Association's program consists of screening for atrial fibrillation with palpitation of the pulse first. If the rhythm is not irregular, the individual is sent to the next station for blood pressure screening. If the pulse is irregular, a modified EKG is performed to rule out atrial fibrillation.

At the blood pressure station the blood pressure is measured in the left arm and recorded. If the pressure is elevated above 140/90, the pressure is also measured in the right arm and recorded. The individual is then directed to the carotid screening station where a stethoscope is used to listen over the carotid arteries for a "bruit." A bruit is a swishing noise in the artery which sometimes occurs with a partial obstruction. If a participant has a bruit, he or she is advised to see his or her physician for further evaluation.

Cholesterol screening is available as an option if desired.

A counselor discusses the results with the participant and suggests medical follow-up when necessary.

The methods used for screening for blood pressure and atrial fibrillation as listed above are satisfactory and easy to perform. However, in the case of screening for carotid stenosis, I prefer ultrasound testing done by a technician with the same certification as the technicians in the X-ray department in your local hospital because ultrasound testing is more accurate. Screening facilities with color flow ultrasound machines usually charge around $35 to $40 for a carotid screening test and provide lectures and educational materials as well.[3] Some hospitals occasionally sponsor free screenings, and some HMOs sponsor them.

The largest screening organization in the United States is Life Line Screening of America which is in twenty states and has been providing screening tests for over six years. The company screens patients for carotid artery disease as well as peripheral arterial insufficiency and abnormal cholesterol. They screen with ultrasound for osteoporosis. They perform a blood test, PSA, which is often elevated in men with carcinoma of the prostate gland. Plans are underway to screen for hypertension and auricular fibrillation. Screenings are often done in community centers or churches; when this is done they usually advertise in the local newspapers. If you wish to find out when a screening is scheduled for your area, you can call the home office of Life Line Screening in Cleveland, Ohio. Their telephone number is 1-800-897-9177. Please refer to the Appendix for an informative interview about Life Line.

Another company actively promoting a screening program is Longevity, Inc. They use a similar abbreviated duplex ultrasound for carotid screening.

Also active in screening for carotid stenosis is the Society for Vascular Technology under the direction of George S.

Lavenson, Jr., M.D. Their program is called the Carotid Artery Risk Factor Ultrasound Study.[4] Dr. Lavenson has published several articles concerning that program. He is a strong advocate for carotid screening. By the time you are reading this book, there will likely be some other screening programs underway.

Screening for Atrial Fibrillation

Screening for atrial fibrillation is not as common as screening for carotid stenosis, but this is almost as important. In order to detect atrial fibrillation, a single-lead electrocardiogram is performed. If the rhythm appears irregular, a physician then studies the tracing to make a decision whether or not atrial fibrillation is present. The person being screened is sent a letter with a picture of the rhythm strip suggesting that he may have atrial fibrillation. The company recommends that he see his physician so that he may have additional testing, with a complete 12-lead electrocardiogram. If, in fact, he has atrial fibrillation, a positive diagnosis can be made, and the patient can either be converted to a normal rhythm or anticoagulation treatment can be instituted.

Screening for Hypertension to Prevent Cerebral Hemorrhage

Hypertension can be screened by simply taking the blood pressure in both arms. Blood pressure is labile or changeable in many individuals, often shifting above normal and below normal many times in the same day. Since the anxiety of having one's pressure taken sometimes causes the pressure to go up, it may be necessary to have the blood pressure taken in both arms on several occasions to establish a suspicion that hypertension exists on a regular basis. If, however, a high blood pressure is obtained on a screening test, then the person would receive a letter that the blood pressure was greater than 140/90 on a particular date. That person can then take the letter to his physician. The physician can make a final decision if hypertension exists and if medication is to be prescribed, or if additional diagnostic studies are indicated to see if the cause of the hypertension can be determined and corrected. In any event, the blood pressure should be brought back to normal levels to prevent arterial damage in many different organs and to prevent stroke. If left untreated, the hypertension can weaken the arteries in the brain and lead to a ruptured blood vessel with hemorrhage into the brain causing stroke. This is one of the mechanisms for the proximate cause of stroke. In addition, hypertension speeds up the atherosclerotic process resulting in the more rapid development of carotid stenosis to cause stroke in the future.

Making the Final Diagnosis

Screening tests do not make the diagnosis but only select people who need to see their doctors because of the likelihood that they have a problem. When a person is found to have a positive screening test for carotid stenosis, atrial fibrillation, or hypertension, the patient receives a letter from the screening company with a copy of the report to take to his physician. The physician will look at the report and decide which additional tests need to be performed in order to make a definitive diagnosis. In the case of carotid stenosis, a Certified Letter would be sent to the person who had the screening if the test showed a moderately severe or severe degree of stenosis in a carotid artery. The doctor would take a history, listen to the carotid arteries with a stethoscope for bruits and then send the patient for additional testing. That additional testing could be either a complete carotid and vertebral color flow ultrasound test at an accredited vascular laboratory, a Magnetic Resonance Angiogram (MRA) of the carotid and vertebral arteries, an intra-arterial digital carotid arteriogram, or an intravenous digital carotid arteriogram. The patient would not need all of these tests, but would probably be well advised to have at least one of them.

What To Do If Atrial Fibrillation Screening Test Is Positive

If the screening test is positive for possible atrial fibrillation, a letter will be received recommending that the person see his physician and take a copy of the report there for review. The physician will likely listen to the heart, collect a complete medical history and do a physical examination to look for signs of congestive heart failure or symptoms of coronary artery disease. He will ask the patient if he feels that his heart has an irregular rhythm or if he can sometimes feel his heart beating or has a sensation almost as though it turned over. Atrial fibrillation is an abnormal rhythm in the upper chambers of the heart. When the upper chambers of the heart beat in this irregular manner, thrombi can form there. The thrombi can often wash up into the brain arteries causing stroke. Atrial fibrillation is thought to be present in two million people in the United States. Clots forming in and embolizing from the heart chambers to the brain in these patients cause about 75,000 strokes per year.

The physician will recommend a complete electrocardiogram to further evaluate the heart, and he may also order an echocardiogram to look for thrombi in the heart chambers. If atrial fibrillation is confirmed with these more sophisticated tests, the physician will likely try, either medically or electrically, to convert the rhythm back to a normal sinus rhythm. If not successful, he will likely order treatment with an anticoagulant medication such as warfarin to help prevent clots from forming.

Sometimes these tests are performed by a family practitioner or internal medicine specialist, but frequently the patient will be referred to a cardiologist to make the definitive diagnosis and commence treatment.

What to do if screening test for hypertension is positive.

In the case of hypertension, the physician would probably have the person come in for a complete physical examination and blood pressure check. He would take the blood pressure or have it taken on several additional occasions before making a diagnosis of hypertension. Additional tests would be performed to try to determine why the patient had hypertension, to determine if it was "essential" hypertension or if it were due to kidney disease or renal artery stenosis. He would also rule out one of the unusual causes for hypertension such as coarctation of the aorta or an adrenal tumor. After other causes were ruled out and if the diagnosis were "essential" hypertension, the physician would likely treat the patient with medication to bring the blood pressure down to normal levels and thereby reduce the risk of stroke and other complications of hypertension. High blood pressure is considered to be a pressure consistently over 140/90 mmHg.

CHAPTER FOUR

Considering Surgery

Referral to a Surgeon

After the medical physician has seen the results of the screening test and ordered the more definitive tests discussed in the previous chapter, he can confirm whether or not significant carotid stenosis is present. The medical doctor will then suggest a referral to a vascular surgeon, cardiovascular surgeon, or neurosurgeon for a consultation to determine if the surgeon agrees that carotid endarterectomy is necessary. If the definitive tests have shown that the degree of carotid stenosis is less than 60 percent and there are no ulcerated plaques visible, then he likely will not have recommended a surgical consultation. If, on the other hand, the definitive tests have shown greater than 60 percent stenosis in a carotid artery, and particularly if there is any evidence to suggest an ulcerated plaque, then a referral to a surgeon experienced in this field is indicated. The question now will be what kind of training for this type of surgery is necessary? What background qualifies a physician to perform this surgery successfully?

When any student graduates from medical school he must decide if he wants to be a family practice physician, or if he wants to enter a different specialty. Each specialty has certain requirements. In the case of surgery, a person must have five years of residency training in a program of gradually increasing responsibility in order to finish and be eligible to take the board examinations for general surgery. The resident learns by rotating through each surgical subspecialty how to be fairly proficient in each field. He will have some training in neurological, orthopedic, and vascular surgery. Most of this training, however, will be in general surgery, including learning to do operations on the stomach, gallbladder, intestines, pancreas, and liver. He will also learn how to perform hernia repairs and remove soft tissue tumors. After completing a residency in general surgery, a physician may decide that he wants further training in one of the subspecialties he practiced briefly in the rotation experience. If he decides he wants to become a vascular surgeon, he will need to take at least one additional year of vascular-surgical training in order to be "board eligible" in vascular surgery. If he wants to become a thoracic or cardiovascular surgeon, he must take at least two additional years of training in thoracic and cardiovascular surgery before becoming board eligible. During that time he will become proficient in operations on the organs in the chest cavity—including the lungs and heart—and all of the major blood vessels in the chest and neck. If he wants to become a neurosurgeon he would take one year of residency in a general surgery program and then switch over to a neurosurgery residency which would require six additional years of training. Upon completion of this program, he would be proficient at operating on the brain and all of the peripheral nerves as well as the arteries supplying the brain.

If a patient is diagnosed as having carotid stenosis and is referred to a surgeon, it should preferably be to a vascular surgeon, a cardiovascular surgeon, or a neurosurgeon.

When the patient arrives with the referral for the consultation, the surgeon will review the patient's history and do a physical examination. He will study the results of the tests which have been obtained by the referring physician. This would include the ultrasound screening test of the carotid arteries, and it would no doubt include a complete carotid and vertebral ultrasound done in an accredited vascular laboratory. Frequently it would also include an intra-arterial digital carotid arteriogram or an MRA of the carotid arteries. It might also include a CT scan or an MRI of the brain.

After the history and physical examination have been completed and the results of the tests reviewed, the surgeon will decide if there are any contraindications to surgery or any extenuating circumstances which would make the operation more dangerous. The surgeon will usually discuss carotid stenosis in detail with the patient, along with his opinion of the risks involved for this particular case. If there are no contraindications, he would probably recommend that the patient proceed with carotid endarterectomy for removal of the blockage from the artery to prevent a stroke from occurring.

The surgeon should discuss the operation with the patient in detail, explaining why he recommends it be done, whether it should be done under local or general anesthesia, and whether any type of monitoring of the brain will be used during the operative procedure to protect the brain from cerebral ischemia or lack of oxygen. If he does not explain all of these things, then it will be necessary for the patient to ask certain questions which appear in "Key Questions to Ask the Surgeon."

Knowing the General Procedures

It is important for the patient to know enough about the operation so that he or she understands what is going to be done in surgery. It is necessary for him or her to cooperate fully, so that the operation can be performed in the safest way. By knowing about the procedure, the patient is able to ask certain questions of the surgeon who is consulting and recommending the operation to determine that he is the right person for the job. While endarterectomy is not a terribly difficult operation, it must be done expeditiously and the brain must be protected at all times during the procedure. The operation is what surgeons call a very "unforgiving" operation in that any minor misjudgment can cause catastrophic complications which cannot be corrected. Since the earliest period of controversy concerning the medical or surgical treatment of this disease, articles appeared in literature written by neurologists claiming that the complication rate of the operation in some cities had been shown to be inordinately high.[1] It has now been proven, in the large, carefully controlled studies, that the operation is superior to medical management for this condition, and that, in the hands of experienced surgeons, the risk is low. The recommended acceptable limits of combined morbidity and mortality due to stroke during or following endarterectomy are shown in figure 4.1. Patients with asymptomatic carotid stenosis should have no more than a 3 percent combined morbidity and mortality. Patients suffering transient ischemic attacks should not have more than a 5 percent combined morbidity and mortality risk. Patients with previous ischemic strokes should expect no more than 7 percent risk, and patients with recurrent carotid stenosis, 7 percent risk. Mortality risk for all groups should not exceed 2 percent.

Patients with asymptomatic carotid stenosis	3 percent
Patients with transient ischemic attacks	5 percent
Patients with history of previous ischemic stroke	7 percent
Patients with recurrent carotid stenosis	7 percent
Mortality for all groups	2 percent

Figure 4.1. Acceptable limits of combined morbidity and mortality during carotid endarterectomy or following the operation within 30 days.

In order to do the operation and maintain a low risk of morbidity and mortality, the surgeon must pay particular attention to detail. While there often exists more than one way to do a thing and get a good result, in the case of this operation it is important that all choices be accurate. When the operation is performed under local anesthesia with an electroencephalogram measuring the activity of the brain waves during the operation, a surgeon can tell instantly if any ischemia or stroke occurs. After doing 7,854 of these operations in that manner, it was possible for me to learn which parts of the procedure were particularly dangerous and prone to cause complications. It was possible then to change the technique in such a way as to reduce the risk.

A description of my preferred operative technique for this procedure is as follows:

The operation can be done safely under general anesthesia or under local anesthesia (cervical block anesthesia). Many surgeons prefer general anesthesia because it is effective, the patients have no anxiety or discomfort, and the anesthesiologist can easily maintain the airway. Some anesthetic agents have a slight brain protective effect during ischemia. The major disadvantage of general anesthesia is that when you put the patient to sleep you lose the very best way of monitoring to be sure there is no cerebral ischemia during the operation.

Fortunately, the operation can also be performed safely under local anesthesia (cervical block anesthesia), which is a sort of "twilight sleep." The patient is sedated, but the area of the operation is anesthetized with local anesthesia similar to that which your dentist uses. When done properly, patients have no discomfort during the operative procedure. They are able to talk and squeeze their contralateral hand to let the surgeon know that they are doing well. And there are additional advantages. A patient under local anesthesia does not get nauseated and does not have labile blood pressure during the operative procedure or after it. The patient goes to the recovery room in an alert state. There is less incidence of respiratory distress, and the patient is usually able to be discharged from the hospital a little sooner than those who have had general anesthesia. Finally, there is less risk of cardiac complications with local anesthesia.

It is important to know more about anesthesia. Chapter Six will go into more detail to explain successful and safe techniques. Many patients and doctors have found that coping with the effects and aftereffects of general anesthesia can be among the most difficult part of the entire procedure, so it is important to become as well informed as possible on this subject.

Electroencephalogram Monitoring During the Operation:

It is not difficult to have an EEG technician perform a continuous 16-channel EEG tracing just prior to the time of the incision for the operation and continue it throughout the operative procedure. The intraoperative interpretation of the brain waves is performed by a registered EEG technician and is officially read by a neurologist postoperatively. In most cases the EEG tracing remains normal throughout the operative procedure; the patient remains alert and able to move his contralateral extremities. If the operation is being done under local anesthesia, the EEG allows more accurate evaluation of the integrity of the brain, insofar as ischemia is concerned. This is an advantage of local rather than general anesthesia. It is a little safer to have local anesthesia in conjunction with an electroencephalogram (EEG). With two methods of monitoring, one is sure that everything is all right. In addition, the EEG shows brain waves on the surface of the brain better than in the deeper areas. Occasionally a patient can have an apparently normal electroencephalogram, but if he is under local anesthesia, he might be unable to speak or move his contralateral extremities. No single monitoring parameter is considered to be totally reliable, so the surgeon should either shunt all patients during carotid endarterectomy or else monitor all patients and promptly shunt those in whom any monitoring parameter indicates ischemia. Data from the Mayo Clinic concerning cerebral ischemia during clamp-off time during carotid endarterectomy indicated that more than 20 percent of patients have significant ischemia during the operative procedure unless a shunt is used. In my personal series of 7,854 procedures done under local anesthesia with EEG, 20 percent required shunts because of ischemia. Most surgeons agree that the safest procedure is for all patients to be shunted or for patients to be monitored and selective shunting carried out on those who have a low stump pressure or abnormal EEG or signs of ischemia if under local anesthesia. It is too much like "Russian roulette" to have this operation done under general anesthesia with no monitoring to test for ischemia of the brain by a surgeon who never shunts. Unfortunately, there are some surgeons who never monitor, never shunt, and still use general anesthesia for the operation.

Use of Occlusion Catheters in the Internal Carotid Artery:

Sometimes the atherosclerotic plaque extends high in the internal carotid artery; even so high that there are reports in the literature about how to dislocate the mandible in order to get to these high lesions. Actually, the use of an occlusion catheter, which is small and easy to work around, allows complete control of back-bleeding from the internal carotid artery. It also allows clear visualization of the end point so these high lesions can be properly managed in a safe and effective way prior to insertion of a shunt without the necessity of dislocating the mandible.

Technique of Carotid Endarterectomy

The patient is taken into the operating room and given intravenous sedation with Versed, which is a sedative. The head is arranged away from the side to be operated on to extend the neck. An incision is made in a skin crease near the anterior border of the long muscle, called the sternocleidomastoid muscle. The incision is carried down to a point just anterior to the internal jugular vein. Care is taken not to injure the mandibular branch of the facial nerve. Branches of the internal jugular vein crossing the carotid artery are ligated. A vessel loop is placed gently around the common carotid artery and sutures of 2.0

CONSIDERING SURGERY

black silk are placed around the external and internal carotid arteries for control. The sutures are used on the internal and external carotid arteries because it takes less manipulation to place the sutures than the vessel loop. It is extremely important not to manipulate the artery at this point because in some cases there are small clots and debris inside the artery which, if agitated, will wash up to the brain causing a stroke before the surgeon even opens the artery. By using the suture technique around the internal and external carotid arteries, one minimizes that risk. The hypoglossal nerve, vagus nerve, superior laryngeal nerve, recurrent laryngeal nerve, and superior thyroid artery are identified and protected. The superior thyroid artery is not ligated either temporarily or permanently. The superior thyroid artery has been found to be an important source of collateral circulation during carotid endarterectomy and must be protected in order to take advantage of that collateral circulation during clamp-off time (see figure 4.2).

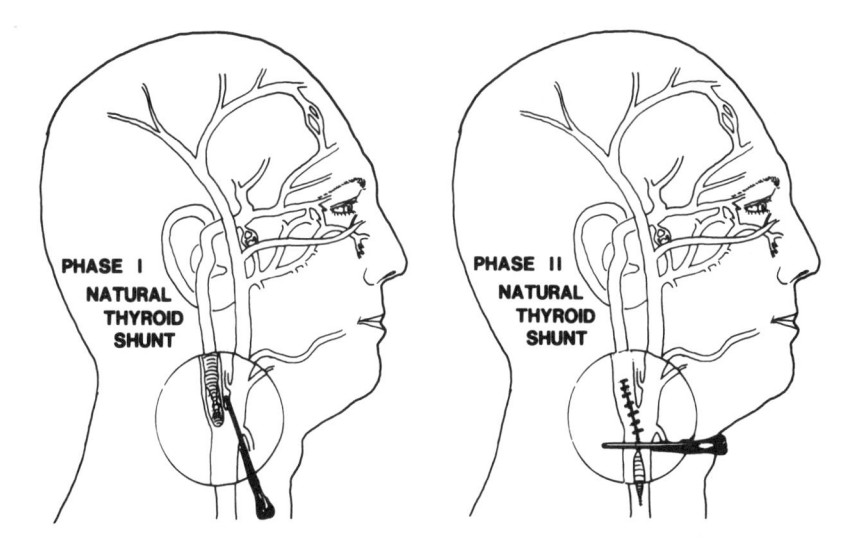

Figure 4.2. Demonstration of arterial clamp positions to take best advantage of collateral circulation to the brain.

Extreme care must be taken to manipulate the carotid artery and its branches as little as possible so as not to dislodge debris from an ulcerated plaque. Ten thousand units of sodium-heparin are given intravenously and after three minutes the surgeon goes through a checklist almost like a pilot before taking off in an airplane.

1. He asks the EEG technician if the electroencephalogram appears normal.
2. He asks the anesthesiologist if the blood pressure is at least as high as the patient's normal blood pressure.
3. He asks the anesthesiologist to confirm patient responses; the anesthesiologist in turn asks the patient to squeeze his contralateral hand, if the operation is being done under local anesthesia, and reports the response.
4. The surgeon asks the anesthesiologist to confirm that the heparin has been given.

If all seems to be in order, the common carotid artery is clamped with a noncrushing arterial clamp and the external carotid artery is clamped with a spring bulldog clamp at an angle, allowing the superior thyroid artery to continue feeding the external carotid artery during clamp-off time to take advantage of the collateral circulation from the superior thyroid artery. This natural collateral circulation through the external carotid artery into the brain helps to reduce the risk of cerebral ischemia during clamp-off time. No clamps are placed on the internal carotid artery. Back-bleeding from the internal carotid is controlled with the loop of 2 "0" silk until an occlusion catheter can be inserted. On one occasion, while I was using clamps instead of occlusion catheters, the patient had an embolus and had a stroke immediately following the application of the clamp on the internal carotid artery and before the artery was even opened. One of the advantages of doing endarterectomy under local anesthesia with EEG control is that complications such as that can be noted immediately and the technique can be changed to prevent future problems.

An arteriotomy incision is made anterolaterally on the common carotid artery extending onto the bulbous portion of the internal carotid artery. A 4 French or 5 French balloon occlusion catheter is then inserted into the internal carotid artery and the balloon is inflated gently with normal saline, with just enough pressure to stop back-bleeding from the internal carotid artery. If there are no EEG or clinical changes of ischemia, and if the stump flow appears adequate, the endarterectomy is completed without the use of an internal carotid shunt. If, however, there are EEG or clinical changes of ischemia, or if the stump pressure does not look vigorous, an internal shunt is inserted adjacent to the occlusion catheter and the occlusion catheter balloon is deflated and removed. A Pruitt-Inahara carotid shunt could be inserted first into the internal carotid or first into the common carotid since the catheter could be flushed out of the side port from either direction to get rid of particles before allowing blood to go to the brain. It is usually preferable to remove much of the plaque, including all ulcerations, prior to insertion of the shunt. The plaque in the internal carotid artery is clearly visible because the occlusion catheter is small and easy to work around and the balloon on the occlusion catheter and on the shunt hold the artery open allowing easy visualization of the end point even with high lesions.

If the plaque is severely adherent or brittle and removal of it appears as though it would take more than four minutes, it would be necessary to extend the arteriotomy incision higher than the distal extent of the plaque so that the shunt can be inserted without fear of getting particles into the shunt itself. A dissector is used to find the appropriate plane for removal of the plaque and the removal is from the most proximal part of the arteriotomy incision in the common carotid, proceeding distally into the external carotid first, and then into the internal carotid artery. Small pickups are used to remove any particles which remain, keeping in mind that the end point in the internal carotid artery is the most important part of the procedure. There is no substitute for an adequate end point! All of the plaque must be removed! If there appears to be any plaque left in the internal carotid it must be removed. If after removal of all of the plaque there remains an intimal flap, the flap should be sutured down. The endarterectomy is not completed until the end point is clean. It should rarely be necessary to place any stitches in the internal carotid at the distal portion of the endarterectomized segment. The distal end ordinarily is quite smooth, with a thin, well-attached intima above.

    The carotid artery is flushed with heparinized saline solution after all plaque has been removed. The balloon from the occlusion catheter holds the artery open so the end point can be carefully visualized. A satisfactory end point is considered to be imperative. The external carotid artery is fully endarterectomized from within until there are no residual plaques or intimal flaps. This part of the procedure is done without making an incision on the external carotid artery. When the endarterectomy is completed the arteriotomy incision is repaired with 5.0 or 6.0 Prolene sutures, beginning at the most cephalad position on the internal carotid artery and extending caudad to a point below the bifurcation. This is important because it allows for the use of collateral circulation. When the arteriotomy incision is closed to an area about 0.5 cm below the bifurcation, the clamp from the external carotid artery is moved to the area just below the bifurcation and the balloon occlusion catheter in the internal carotid artery is removed. This change in position of the bulldog clamp allows an increased amount of collateral circulation to go to the brain in cases where no internal shunt is being used. Flow from the branches of the external carotid artery will now supply the internal carotid artery and there are very few patients who have any ischemia with this configuration. This part has been termed the "Second phase of the natural thyroid shunt," recognizing that much of this collateral circulation comes from the superior thyroid artery (see figure 2.1). A second suture of 5.0 or 6.0 Prolene is then begun on the proximal portion of the common carotid artery incision and sutured up to the first stitch, at which time flushing is carried out from the common carotid artery and then from the external and internal carotid arteries before placing the last few stitches in the common carotid incision. Blood is allowed to flow first through the external carotid and then through the internal carotid, so that any debris or air is flushed into the face and scalp vessels, rather than into the internal carotid which goes to the brain. The patient is given 50 mg of protamine sulfate to partially reverse the heparin.

In cases where a shunt has been used, the arteriotomy is done in the same manner, and the shunt is removed before placing the last two stitches. The artery is examined with a sterile Doppler or ultrasound to listen for a high pitch or to see any residual plaque or intimal flap. If the pulsation in the internal carotid artery feels normal and there are no thrills, the procedure is completed. If after closure, however, the flow does not feel adequate, or if there is a palpable thrill or the Doppler or ultrasound are not normal, then it is necessary to re-clamp the common carotid artery and the external carotid artery as before to reopen the artery and examine carefully for technical errors. If the artery is reopened, a patch graft is sutured onto the site of the arteriotomy incision to increase the size of the vessel. This is occasionally necessary.

Patients are given small additional amounts of heparin over the ensuing twenty hours in an effort to prevent the formation of thrombi on the raw surface where the endarterectomy has been performed. Postoperatively the blood pressure is carefully monitored in the recovery room and in the Intensive Care Unit, and the patients are observed for cardiac arrhythmias, respiratory disturbances, seizures, TIAs, or stroke.

Patches are liberally used in patients with small arteries, in all cases of recurrent carotid stenosis, and in those patients who have turbulence inside the vessel at the termination of the procedure. When in doubt, it is best to use a patch graft. Some surgeons prefer to patch almost all of them.

Carotid Endarterectemy Dissectors

Carotid endarterectomy is a procedure which should be done as expeditiously as possible to minimize cerebral ischemia. Having the proper tools at hand for performing the procedure helps facilitate the dissection and prevent complications. Most surgeons perform this operation with elevators or dissectors. These elevators are provided by the nurse on the Mayo Table, and are used for separating the plaque from the normal wall of the artery. The tools to be used are most often selected by the circulating nurse from a shelf of instruments. Dissectors for carotid endarterectomy should be chosen with care because each dissector has a specific function for making the operation progress rapidly without problems.

A carotid endarterectomy dissector kit is often prepared iscluding five dissectors (see figure 4.3). The dissector labeled "a" is a standard Freer elevator, which is currently available in almost all operating rooms and which is used for separating the plaque from the residual soft media of the vessel up to an area about 0.5 cm above the bifurcation into the internal and external carotid arteries.

The dissector labeled "b" is a straight dissector, smaller at the distal end for use in the internal and external carotid arteries where the vessel is smaller. The dissectors are to be used

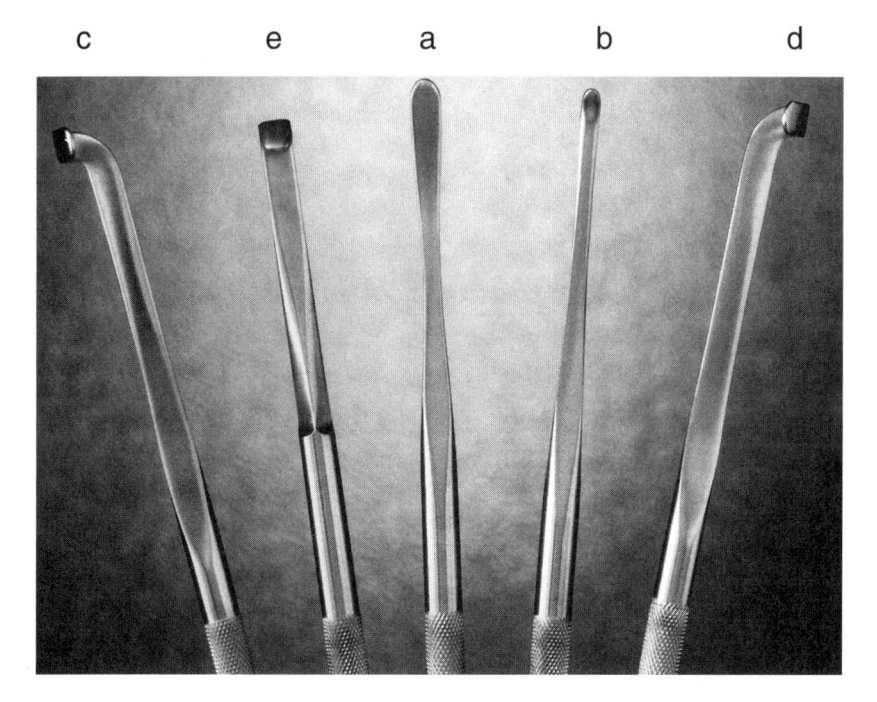

Figure 4.3. Dissector kit with five dissectors used during carotid endarterectomy. Each dissector is designed to help perform a specific part of the operation.

to separate the plaque from the residual soft media as high as the plaque extends.

The dissector labeled "c" is one with a curved distal end slightly tilted externally at its tip, which is used to separate the plaque from the residual soft media from the bifurcation down into the proximal part of the common carotid artery. This dissector is especially designed for use in the part of the common carotid artery which is lying across from the surgeon using the device to separate the plaque from the normal arterial wall.

The dissector labeled "d" is a mirror image of the dissector labeled "c" described above and is to be used to separate the plaque from the soft media. It is very good for separating plaque and forming a line of dissection in the vessel wall proximal to the surgeon who is using the instrument. Use of this device helps to prevent inadvertent puncture wounds in the posterior wall of the vessel caused by trying to use a right angle for this part of the procedure.

The dissector labeled "e" is a dissector which is shaped like a right angle but has a flattened tip to keep it from puncturing the posterior wall of the proximal carotid artery near the area where the plaque is to be divided for removal.

In performing a carotid endarterectomy procedure, the surgeon will find that the plaque often extends down the common carotid for quite a distance, sometimes down to the level of the clavicle. This plaque often is not large enough to be obstructing and not large enough to warrant opening the artery that far down for its removal because in doing so one would likely get more stenosis of the common carotid artery as a result of the procedure. The common practice is to divide the proximal part of the plaque several centimeters below the bifurcation. It is important that this be a neat division of the plaque so that no particles will be remaining which could cause an embolus. There is not another dissector available which is shaped properly for the inferior separation of this plaque, allowing for it to be removed expeditiously in a neat manner for prevention of small particle embolization. Some surgeons use a right angle clamp for doing this inferior portion of the endarterectomy, and in cases where the plaque is stuck tightly to the posterior wall, the sharp point of the right angle clamp sometimes penetrates the common carotid wall, requiring suturing with multiple small stitches. In order to avoid this complication and to make the operation easier, dissector "e" was designed and is commercially available. It helps to prevent damage to the posterior wall of the media. With this device the plaque can be lifted from the media circumferentially and proximally without penetrating the posterior wall of the common carotid artery, and the proximal portion of the plaque can be divided without leaving particles which could embolize.

In order to perform carotid endarterectomy with a minimum of risk, careful attention must be paid to a long list of items, including the following:

1. Proper selection of patients
2. Timing of the operation
3. Preoperative preparation of the patient to be sure that cardiac and respiratory status are okay for surgery
4. Selection of anesthesia appropriate for the patient
5. Maintenance of adequate blood pressure and prevention of arrhythmias
6. Avoidance of manipulation of the vessels during dissection; consider using loops of sutures instead of vessel loops for control
7. Avoidance of placing clamps on internal carotid artery

8. Completion of surgical checklist before clamping off vessels
9. Avoidance of occlusion of superior thyroid artery so that it can be used for collateral
10. Monitoring of more than one parameter during the procedure to avoid cerebral ischemia and shunting when necessary, preferably with a balloon shunt
11. Utilization of a balloon occlusion catheter in the common carotid artery before the balloon shunt is used so that the end point can be seen better
12. Forward and back flushing of the shunt through a side port before allowing blood to go to the brain
13. Removal of all the plaque including the loose circular fibers of the media
14. Placement of the incision in the common and internal carotid arteries in an anterolateral position
15. Avoidance of making incision on internal carotid artery too high
16. Usage of proper tools for the procedure; specific dissectors or elevators are important
17. Utilization of patch graft when internal carotid artery appears small or when endarterectomy site is rough
18. Adequate flushing to prevent emboli
19. Evacuation of blood through external carotid before internal carotid at the end of the procedure
20. Maintenance of low-dose heparin therapy for the first twenty-four hours following surgery to prevent small thrombi from forming on the raw endarterectomized segment of the artery

21. Monitoring of patient postoperatively for arrhythmias, hypotension, or severe hypertension

Most surgeons who are experienced in carotid endarterectomy surgery are aware of the items mentioned above and will be paying close attention to all of these details. If, however, you determine at your preoperative visit that you are with one of the surgeons who, in your opinion, is not going to be paying attention to all of these, then perhaps a different referral from your medical physician would be indicated.

Figure 4.4.
A calcific plaque with multiple ulcerations causing 80% obstruction of internal carotid artery. This patient had a loud, high-pitched bruit over the artery but was asymptomatic.

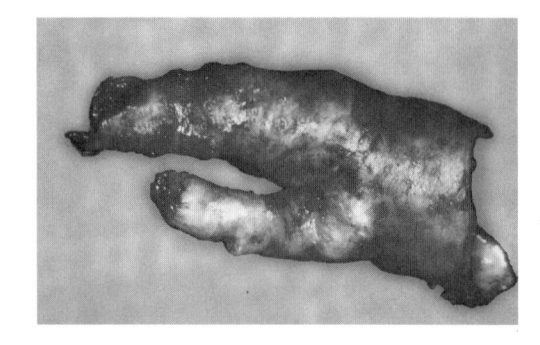

Figure 4.5.
A rubbery plaque involving the bifurcation of the left carotid artery demonstrating 60% obstruction with ulcerations. This patient had an episode of loss of vision in his left eye.

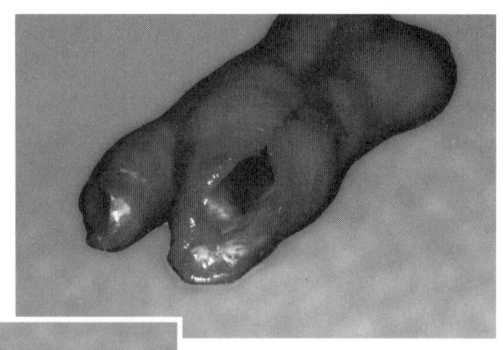

Figure 4.6.
A tight 90% stenosis of internal carotid artery caused by a hard plaque consisting of calcium and cholesterol. This patient was not yet symptomatic, but if left untreated the first symptom might have been a permanent stroke.

Figure 4.7.
A markedly irregular rough and ulcerated plaque causing 70% obstruction of the carotid artery. The patient was symptomatic having intermittent slurring of speech and loss of coordination in the right arm.

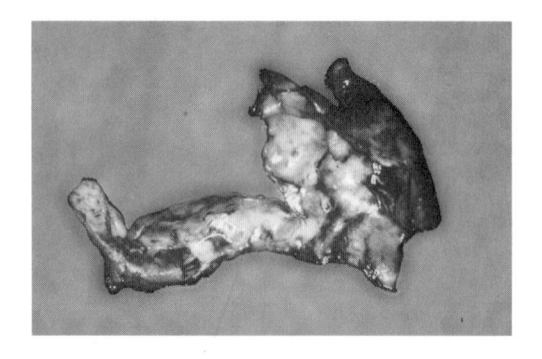

CONSIDERING SURGERY 65

Figure 4.8.
Two pieces of atherosclerotic plaque removed from a carotid artery. The patient was having recurrent TIAs involving confusion and inability to speak clearly. The TIAs stopped after surgical removal of the plaque which was causing 60 percent stenosis.

Figure 4.9.
80% obstruction of an internal carotid artery with ulcerated plaque. This patient had a bruit but was asymptomatic.

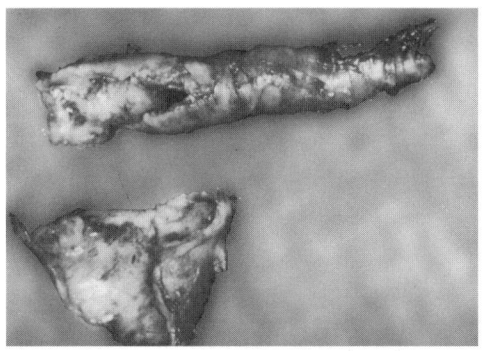

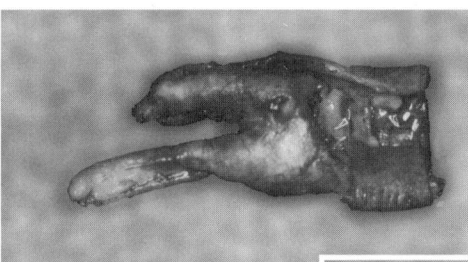

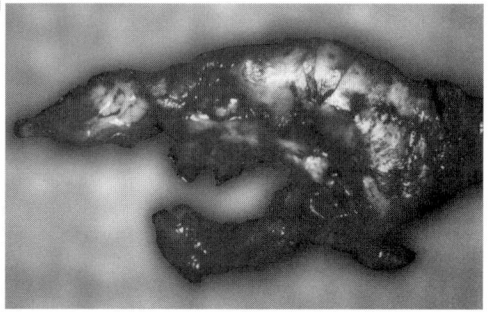

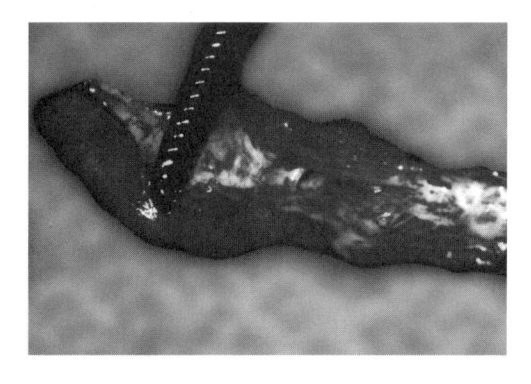

Figure 4.10.
Calcified plaque causing 95% obstruction of internal carotid artery in an asymptomatic person. No bruit was audible.

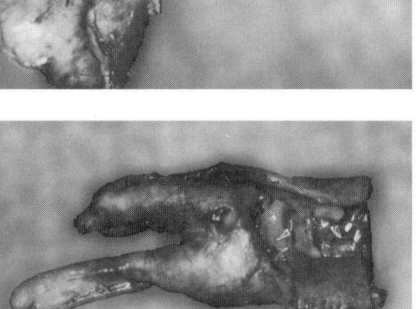

Figure 4.11.
Plaque causing a 70% obstruction removed from a carotid artery of a fifty-year-old man who had recently recovered from a small stroke. If the obstruction had not been removed, he would have been at risk for another stroke in the near future.

CHAPTER FIVE

Seeking Information

Key Questions to Ask the Surgeon

Surgeons who are experienced in carotid endarterectomy procedures are aware of all of the items mentioned in the earlier chapters. If the surgeon you have been referred to fails to discuss the procedure in enough detail for you to be sure of his proficiency, consider asking him or her some of these questions.

1. Are you board certified in your specialty?

Most surgeons are very proud of their qualifications and will be happy to discuss them with you. If you are in the office of a vascular surgeon or a thoracic and cardiovascular surgeon, he should be board certified in his specialty. If you are in the office of a neurosurgeon, he should be board certified in neurosurgery. If he is board certified, it means that he has successfully completed a difficult prescribed program of training in that specialty with a graduated increase in responsibility. After having completed the training program, he successfully passed an examination. This is not to say that there are not many surgeons out there who are not board certified who are fully capable of doing the operation. However, if you are in the office of a board certified surgeon in one of these three specialties, he or she probably is well-trained to do the operation in a credible manner with acceptable risk.

2. Do you do carotid endarterectomy operations frequently?

The answer to this question should be "yes."

3. Have you done this operation more than thirty times?

If he hedged in the answer to question two at all, you must be alert and ask if he or she has done this more than thirty times. The operation requires a great many decisions to be made quickly. Each case is slightly different so that the more experience a surgeon has the better qualified he is to do the surgery safely.

4. Which hospital do you prefer for this operation?

Surgeons often have a preference for a certain hospital for a particular operation. The surgeon might prefer the anesthesiologists, the EEG technicians, or the nursing assistants in the operating room in one hospital over others. Try to accept the hospital recommended by the surgeon rather than forcing your preference on him. If the surgeon feels more comfortable doing this procedure in hospital A instead of hospital B, he probably has a good reason and you should go along with his recommendation if at all possible. The surgeon needs to be comfortable doing the procedure in the hospital chosen. You would not want to be the first case that surgeon has ever done in that particular operating room.

5. What type of anesthesia will you use on me?

Either general anesthesia or sedation plus local anesthesia (cervical block anesthesia) is satisfactory for the operation. If, however, he says that he will use general anesthesia, then it is easily apparent that he will not be able to tell if your brain is getting adequate blood supply during clamp-off time unless some sort of monitoring is being done. If he chooses local anesthesia, then he will be able to tell if the brain is getting enough blood by talking to you or asking you to squeeze your contralateral hand during the operative procedure.

6. Will you use a shunt for the operation during clamp-off time?

If he says "maybe," ask how will he tell if you need a shunt? How will he tell if your brain is getting enough blood while the artery is clamped off? These are questions that need to be answered in advance. You do not want a surgeon doing this operation who is unsure about when he or she is going to use a shunt or under what circumstances he will use one. You want a surgeon who has decided the parameters in advance and knows under what circumstances he will shunt and will not shunt, and, if he will shunt, which shunt he will use and whether or not he is proficient with the use of that shunt.

The methods of monitoring the brain to decide if a shunt is necessary or not include:

1. Talking to a patient who is under local anesthesia and

asking him to perform minor tasks such as squeezing his contralateral hand or counting to three

2. EEG done during the procedure to monitor the brain waves which will develop loss of amplitude and slowing if the brain is not getting enough blood during clamp-off time

3. Measurement of stump pressure or back-bleeding pressure from the internal carotid artery

4. Transcranial Doppler

5. Radioactive Xenon

All of the above methods of monitoring are satisfactory and it is probably best to choose a surgeon who monitors by using at least one of the above. Two methods of monitoring would be better, but at least one is necessary, particularly if the surgeon intends to use general endotracheal anesthesia. If sedation and local anesthesia are chosen, then the surgeon will be able to evaluate the adequacy of collateral circulation to the brain by talking to the patient. In that case, no other monitoring is absolutely necessary, although EEG in conjunction with local anesthesia is a good back-up plan for additional monitoring.

7. Do you use monitoring?

Does the surgeon routinely use EEG monitoring whether he does this operation under general or local anesthesia? If he does, he probably is a very meticulous surgeon who will likely be acutely aware of the adequacy of blood supply to the brain during the procedure. EEG monitoring is readily done and helps in many ways. The EEG technician puts the EEG wires on the scalp prior to the procedure when the patient is in the holding area just before surgery. It is helpful to have an EEG tracing showing the status of the brain waves printed out a few minutes before the operation begins and constantly during the operative procedure. If any type of emergency occurs during the operation, the EEG technician frequently will recognize it first. If there is ischemia to the brain when the carotid artery is clamped off, the EEG technician can notify the surgeon—usually within thirty seconds—allowing him plenty of time to get a shunt in place before brain damage occurs. If the blood pressure drops for any cause, the EEG technologist frequently will notice the change in brain waves first and notify the surgeon and anesthesiologist of the change. If a cardiac arrhythmia develops, the EEG technologist frequently will pick it up first. If cardiac arrest occurs, the EEG technologist many times will detect it before it is noticed by anyone else in the operating room. I feel that EEG monitoring is quite helpful.

8. Do you use any other type of monitoring besides EEG?

The other types of monitoring include measurement of the stump pressure, which is the pressure in the internal carotid artery after the common carotid and the external carotid arteries have been clamped. If the stump pressure is more than 50 millimeters of mercury, then usually, but not always, the patient has enough collateral circulation to the brain so that an internal shunt is not necessary during the procedure. Other methods of monitoring include radioactive Xenon, which is capable of telling the surgeon if the collateral circulation to the brain is adequate. However, this requires considerable equipment which is not available in most hospitals. The transcranial Doppler is a satisfactory monitoring method and can be a great help in deciding on the necessity for an internal shunt. The transcranial Doppler method, however, requires the transcranial Doppler probe to be at an exact angle which must not be disturbed during the operative procedure. That is quite difficult to do, and if transcranial Doppler is the only method of monitoring, you should be sure that the surgeon has used this method on a number of occasions and has worked out the problems of keeping the probe from being disturbed from its proper position during the procedure.

9. If the operation is under local anesthesia, does the anesthesiologist sedate me well before injecting the local anesthesia?

Local anesthesia is a wonderful way of doing this operation. However, some anesthesiologists seem more proficient at the cervical block procedure than others. There is a learning curve. The anesthesiologist should sedate the patient with intravenous sedation prior to injecting the needles for the local anesthesia or cervical block anesthesia. When this procedure is perfected by an anesthesiologist, he can, within five minutes, completely anesthetize the area of the neck where the operation is to be performed so that the patient has absolutely no pain during the operative procedure and the brain can be carefully monitored. For a complete description of the proper method of performing the cervical block anesthesia, please see Chapter Six.

10. If you use local anesthesia, do you also monitor the brain with EEG during the procedure?

It is very desirable to monitor the brain waves with EEG even when local anesthesia is to be used. It is not absolutely necessary, but it still is quite helpful for the value of the EEG and for the other reasons mentioned above. It is very important for the brain to receive adequate oxygen during the time the carotid artery is clamped off. It is the responsibility of the surgeon to see that there is enough cerebral perfusion all during the operation so that the patient will not have a stroke and will be at least as smart after the operation as he was before. Using the EEG as an additional monitoring method helps the surgeon reach that goal. Some physicians will insist that it is an unnecessary, additional procedure and that it increases the cost of the operation, but I feel that it is well worth the additional time and expense for the increase in safety that it provides.

11. How do you feel about using shunts during the operation?

If the surgeon replies that he "never shunts," it is probably best if you thank him for his time and advice, but return to your medical physician and ask for another referral. If he says that he "sometimes shunts," ask him how he decides which patients to shunt and which patients not to shunt. Be certain he has a definite plan for some type of monitoring to be done and that he will make his decision about whether to shunt or not to shunt depending upon the results of the monitoring technique. If he says he uses local anesthesia and shunts those people who quickly go to sleep after the common carotid artery is clamped and/or those who lose the ability to talk or squeeze their contralateral hand, then that is an acceptable plan. Under local anesthetic, as soon as the shunt is in place, the patient will rapidly awake and again be able to talk and squeeze his or her contralateral hand. Actually, if the brain is not getting enough blood, the patient will usually go into a deep sleep within thirty seconds of clamp-off time and if he is in the process of counting to ten, he will say "one, two, three, four," and then go to sleep. Then when the shunt is put into place, he will wake back up and say "five, six, seven, eight," as though he has never been asleep. Remember, the word carotid is derived from a Greek word meaning "to plunge into sleep or stupor," and it was long thought that compressing these arteries would cause unconsciousness. Patients who go to "sleep" during carotid artery procedures do seem to lose consciousness in an unusual way. By doing this operation under local anesthesia, the surgeon has a very good method of monitoring the circulation in the brain and being sure that it is adequate so that the patient does not accidentally drift off into a dangerous "sleep" without its being noticed. If the surgeon uses this as the method of monitoring, it is satisfactory to stay with this surgeon. It is even better to also use EEG to give additional monitoring information which is helpful because in a few cases a patient will get very drowsy from the preoperative medication or sedation, plus some absorption of the local anesthesia, so that evaluating the patient's neurological status can be a little difficult. If the EEG is also present and the brain waves are normal, this is additional assurance that everything is all right and a shunt is not necessary. If the patient becomes quite drowsy and the EEG becomes abnormal, then it is additional evidence that it is necessary to insert a shunt. In addition, the other advantages of the EEG are that the EEG technician frequently will pick up drops in blood pressure or cardiac arrhythmias before the surgeon or anesthesiologist notice the changes.

12. If you use general anesthesia, do you also monitor with EEG and use a shunt?

If the surgeon says he uses general anesthesia and monitors with EEG and uses a shunt on those who have changes of ischemia in the EEG, then stay with this surgeon. That is a satisfactory way of doing it. A physician who says he puts all of his patients to sleep but who also uses shunts with all of them is following an acceptable procedure. If all patients are going to be shunted it is not absolutely necessary that any type of special brain monitoring be done. The EEG would be helpful in letting him know that the shunt is functioning properly and the brain is getting enough blood, and it would also help him to be sure that the blood pressure has not dropped and no arrhythmias have occurred, but it is not absolutely necessary. If he says he just sort of decides during the operation if he thinks a shunt is necessary but does not have a specific monitoring plan and just looks at the carotid pressure from the internal carotid and considers the history and decides whether to shunt, I would not be happy. This is not a good way of deciding who needs a shunt and probably it would be best to leave and thank him for his time. Ask your referring doctor to recommend another surgeon.

If the physician you are considering using says he shunts those who need it, but less than 5 percent need a shunt, then that would be a worrisome statement. We know that cerebral ischemia has been studied extensively, and these studies show that when the common carotid and external carotid are clamped, cerebral ischemia will occur in at least 20 percent of patients. Not all of these patients would get a paralytic stroke if not shunted, but it is not possible to predict which ones will and which ones will not. So, in order to be safe, it is necessary to be liberal enough about the monitoring end points so that a shunt will be used in a minimum of about 15 percent to 20 percent of cases. If a surgeon says that he uses a shunt in less than 5 percent of the cases, things don't add up quite right, so it is probably best to ask your referring doctor for another referral. If he says that he monitors the patient by one of the above methods and uses an internal shunt in 15 percent to 20 percent or more, then stay with this surgeon.

13. Which shunt do you prefer? How long have you used it, and what are the advantages of that shunt?

A shunt is a plastic tube which is used to direct blood around an arteriotomy site, from the common carotid to the internal carotid artery while carotid endarterectomy is being carried out. There are at the present time seven different types available on the market: (1) the Sundt shunt, (2) the Javid shunt, (3) the Brener shunt, (4) the Pruitt-Inahara shunt, (5) the Inahara-Pruitt shunt, (6) the Loftus shunt, and (7) the Argyle shunt. The advantages and disadvantages of each of these shunts are listed underneath the pictures of the shunts (see figures 5.1, 5.2, 5.3, 5.4, 5.5, 5.6, and 5.7).

14. Do you like to use a shunt with or without a side port?

If he or she uses a shunt without a side port, getting rid of air bubbles and calcium can be a problem. How can he be sure that he has gotten out all of the air bubbles and calcium particles if no side port is available to flush them out? If a shunt does not have a side port and a particle gets into the shunt when it is inserted, the only place for that particle to go is to

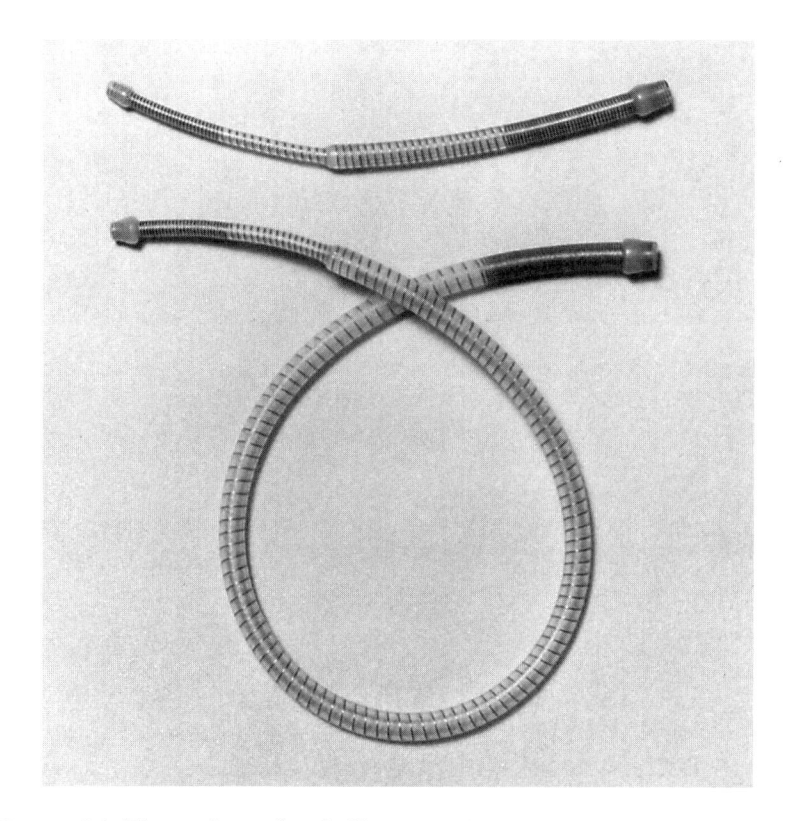

Figure 5.1. The outlying Sundt Shunt is a 30 cm wire-reinforced straight plastic tube without a side port. It has soft, molded tips to reduce trauma to the vessel. It is held in place with tapes. It has a good flow rate. It cannot be clamped without damage to the shunt. An inlying Sundt Shunt is also available which is 10 cm in length. (Photo courtesy of the Heyer-Schulte Company, Goleta, Calif.)

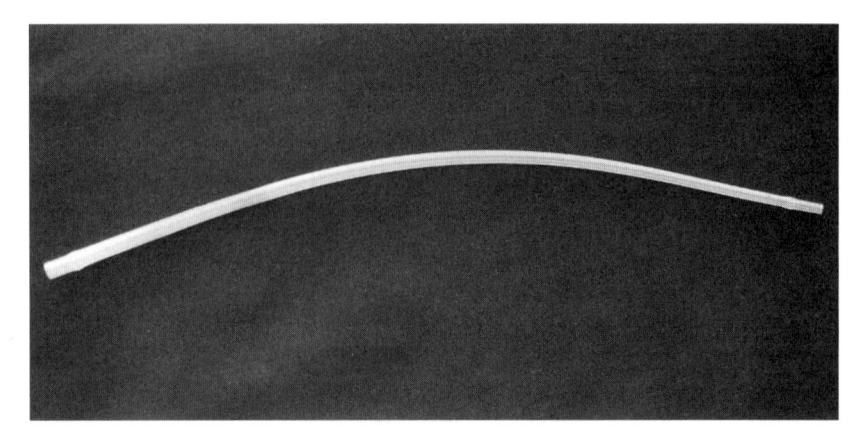

Figure 5.2. The Javid Shunt. This shunt is held in place with metal clamps. There is no side port to get rid of air or particles. It has a good flow rate. (Photo courtesy of Kimberly Caminiti)

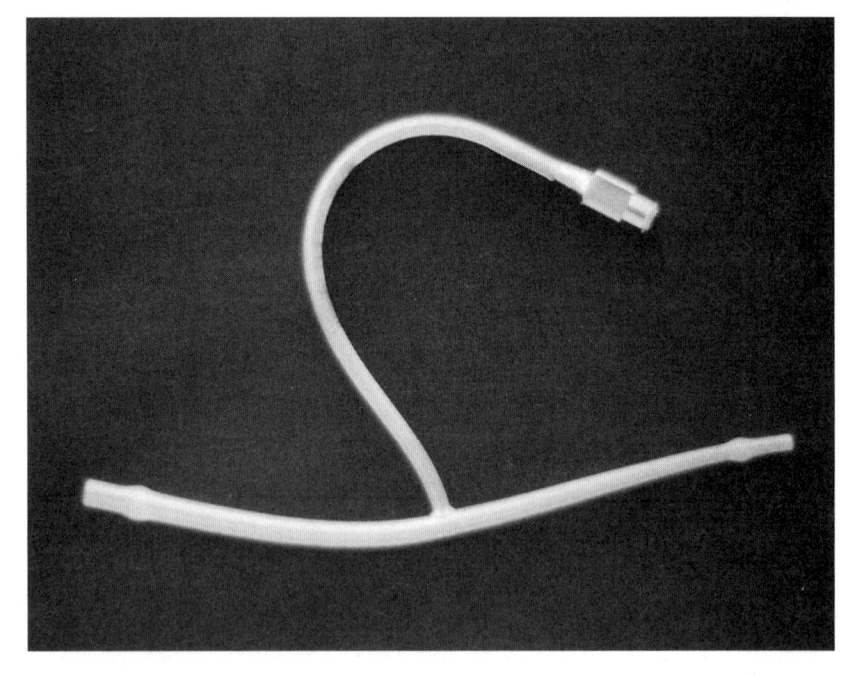

Figure 5.3. The Brener Shunt. Similar to the Javid shunt, this design has the added advantage of a side port. It is held in place with metal clamps. (Photo courtesy of Kimberly Caminiti)

KEY QUESTIONS TO ASK THE SURGEON 79

the brain, which will cause a stroke. Therefore, it is because of this that shunts can sometimes cause strokes. It, therefore, is best to use a shunt with a side port. In addition, a shunt that has a side port can be used to "troubleshoot," to be sure that blood is still going through the shunt while it is in place, rather than just sitting stagnant in the shunt. A side port also helps to be sure that the blood pressure is adequate and that there are no arrhythmias. If a shunt does not have a side port, then once it is in place the surgeon can see the red blood inside of it but cannot tell if that blood is moving or staying still. If a side port is present, he can turn the stop cock and see the flow, reassuring himself that the shunt is working properly. In addition, if there are any changes in the monitoring, the surgeon can open the stop cock and see that the flow is adequate

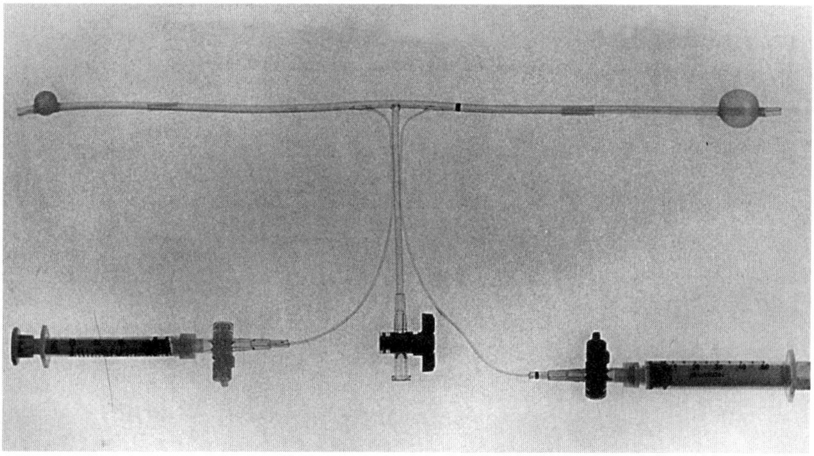

Figure 5.4. The Pruitt-Inahara Shunt is an outlying polyurethane plastic shunt 9 French in diameter and 30 cm in length. The shunt is held in place with balloons. It is provided with or without a side port. It is easy to work around. It has good flow. The balloons hold the internal carotid artery open providing good visibility of the inside of the arteries.(Photo courtesy of Horizon Medical Products, Manchester, Ga.)

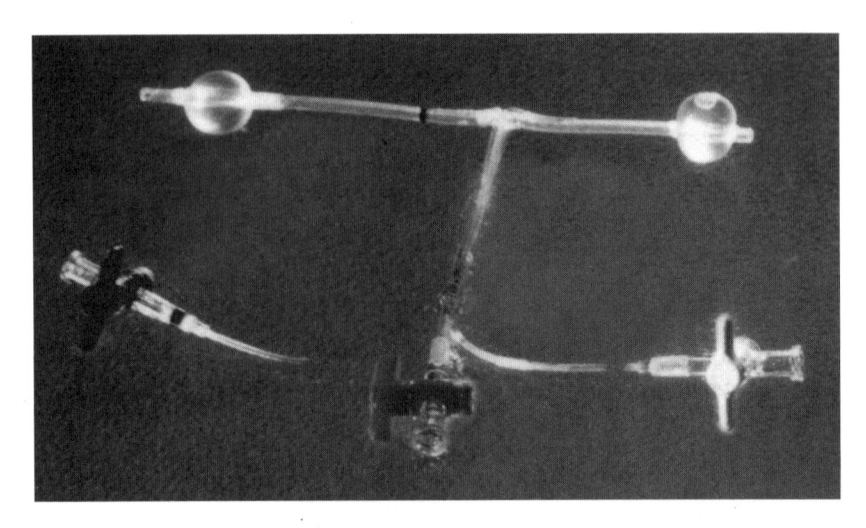

Figure 5.5A. The Inahara-Pruitt Shunt is an inlying Polyurethane shunt that comes with or without a side port. It has an excellent flow rate. It is held in position with balloons. It has a diameter of 9 French and is 15 cm long. It may be clamped without damage to the shunt.

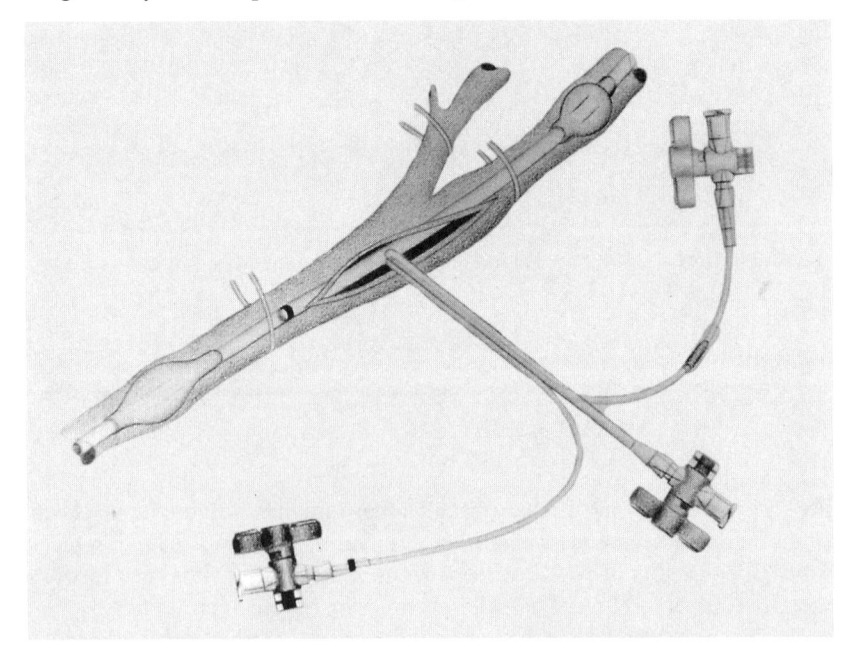

Figure 5.5B. This drawing indicates how the Inahara-Pruitt Shunt is placed in position.(Photos courtesy of Ideas for Medicine, St. Petersburg, Fla.)

KEY QUESTIONS TO ASK THE SURGEON 81

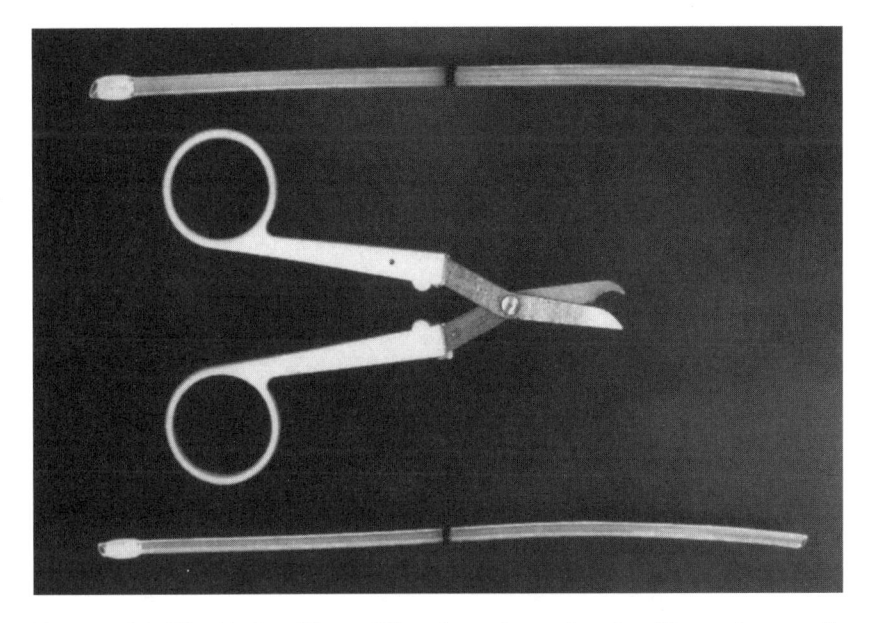

Figure 5.6. The Loftus Shunt. This shunt is made of a silicone isomer. It was developed by Dr. C. M. Loftus. It may be cross-clamped gently with an atraumatic clamp without affecting flow when clamp is removed. The proximal end is held in the artery by a Rummel tourniquet. Two sizes are available. The smaller size is 15 cm in length and has an inside diameter of 2.5 mm. The larger size is 15 cm in length and has an internal diameter of 3.3 mm. There is no side port on this shunt. (Photo courtesy of Heyer-Schulte Company, Goleta, Calif.)

from both directions, proximal and distal, and can notice the forcefulness of the blood coming out of the side port, which is a reflection of the blood pressure. He can also notice the rhythm of the pulse coming out of the side port to be sure there is no arrhythmia. All of these things are helpful, in addition to the fact that the side port allows flushing out of particles and air bubbles before blood flows to the brain. Certainly, a side port is a useful part of a carotid shunt, and you would prefer to use a surgeon who takes advantage of that technology.

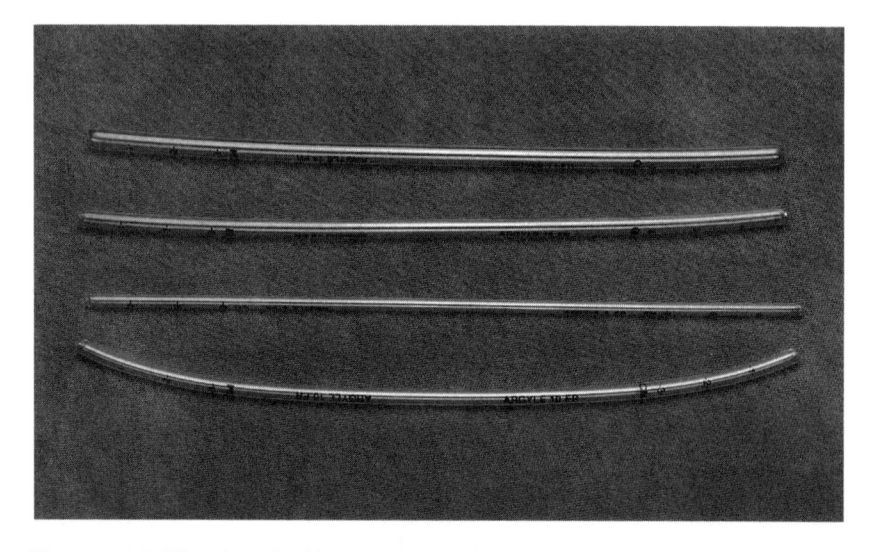

Figure 5.7. The Argyle Shunt. The Argyle Shunt is a polyvinyl chloride shunt which comes in 6F, 8F, 10F, and 14F sizes. It does not have a side port. It is held in place with tapes. The flow rate varies depending on the French size of the shunt. The shunt length is 15 cm. There is an X-ray opaque sentinel line on the shunt. (Photo by Zebra Color, Inc., St. Petersburg, Fla.)

15. Have you tried a shunt with balloons to hold the shunt in place?

Does the surgeon think that balloons would be less traumatic to the lining of the artery than clamps or tourniquets to hold the shunt in place? Five of the shunts listed above are held in place by clamps or tourniquets which pinch the arterial wall against the plastic tubing of the shunt. This tight tourniquet or metal clamp sometimes injures the intima of the artery, and, in the case of the internal carotid artery, the injury might be at a site that the surgeon will never be able to see, so an intimal flap could occur which would later be responsible for a complication. The balloon method of holding the shunt is less traumatic and serves the same purpose.

16. How can you see the end point if the shunt is held in place with a clamp or a tourniquet?

When the shunt is held in place by clamps or tourniquets, the arterial wall is pinched against the plastic tubing, making it impossible to see the area just below and at the level of the clamp or tourniquet. This sometimes causes injury which will not be visualized by the surgeon and loose fragments of plaque can be flushed into the brain after the operation is completed, causing disastrous results. Adequate visualization and management of the end point is the most crucial part of a carotid endarterectomy procedure. Balloon shunts and occlusion catheters help to solve the problem of visualization in high lesions. A balloon in the internal carotid artery holds the vessels open, allowing clear visualization of the end point up inside the artery for several centimeters. The plaque can be removed even above the extent of the arteriotomy incision, shortening the procedure and helping to prevent postoperative re-stenosis. When one uses a balloon shunt it is almost never necessary to suture down the end point in the internal carotid because all of the plaque can be removed regardless of how high the lesion extends. When an internal shunt is not used, an occlusion catheter may be employed in the internal carotid artery. The occlusion catheter is small (only 4 or 5 French), is easy to work around, and allows clear visualization of the end point. The end point is not as clearly visible when an arterial clamp is used. The amount of additional plaque which is removable by this technique is remarkable. See Figure 5.8.

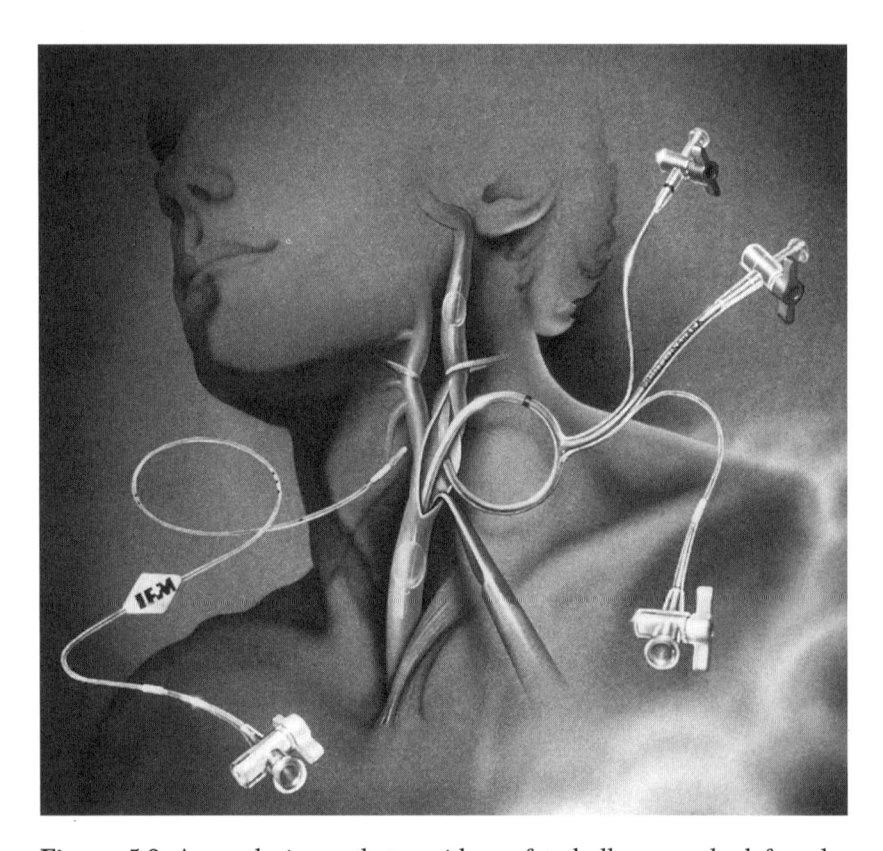

Figure 5.8. An occlusion catheter with a safety balloon on the left and a Model 400–40 Pruitt-Inahara carotid shunt in the left carotid artery of the patient. The smaller occlusion catheter is used in the internal carotid artery before the shunt is inserted because it is atraumatic and easy to work around for removal of high lesions and allows good visualization of the end point. (Photo courtesy of Ideas for Medicine, St. Petersburg, Fla.)

17. How can you be sure the end point is stable and firmly attached to the wall of the vessel so that it will not curl up and obstruct after the operation has been completed?

The intima in the internal carotid artery sometimes is not as firmly attached to the wall of the artery as would be desirable. When no more pieces appear after all of the plaque has been removed, then it is time to sew the artery back up again. However, in truth, there often is some residual loose intima within normal-appearing internal carotid arteries that will lift itself from the media with minimal pressure. If this is not removed it may allow blood to dissect underneath it causing it to curl up and obstruct the lumen of the internal carotid artery. Most vascular surgeons are aware of this danger and will be sure that the intima left behind is firmly attached before closing the arteriotomy incision.

18. Do you remove all of the plaque up in the internal carotid artery, or do you sometimes divide the plaque after taking out most of it, and suture down the end point distally.

Ideally, the surgeon should try to remove all of the atherosclerotic plaque so that no sutures of the intima to the arterial wall are necessary. If there is anything left to sew down, then all of the plaque has not been removed. Any plaque left behind in the internal carotid artery could be undermined by the flow of blood toward the brain, causing particles to be dislodged or allowing the plaque which has been left behind to curl up and obstruct the internal carotid artery. In addition, any plaque left behind could form a basis for plaque to grow again, causing a carotid re-stenosis in a relatively short period of time.

19. Do you agree that the management of the end point is one of the most important parts of this operation.

He should always meticulously prove to himself that the entire plaque has been removed and that the intima left behind is firmly attached to the arterial wall. After all of the atherosclerotic plaque has been removed, if there is an intimal tissue flap it should be sutured down.

20. Do you usually make the incision on the internal carotid artery up to a point above the plaque, or does the incision stop while still on the bulbous portion of the internal carotid artery?

The internal carotid artery gets smaller, the higher above the bifurcation it goes. Sometimes when a carotid endarterectomy is performed, the plaque extends way up on the internal carotid artery where it is very small. If the incision involves this area, the vessel is made smaller by the suturing process, and then, as the artery heals, it retracts and gets even smaller so that one can end up with as much stenosis as was present prior to surgery unless steps are taken to prevent that result. There are two possible ways of handling this problem. The first one is that the surgeon can stop the incision while still on the bulbous, or larger portion of the internal carotid artery, which is sometimes below the actual end point of the plaque. If the surgeon is working with an occlusion catheter or balloon shunt, the balloon will hold the artery open so that the surgeon can remove all of the plaque and see the end point adequately in spite of the fact that the incision is below the region of the end point. There is no substitute for having a perfect end point! The surgeon must cut the internal carotid artery high enough so that he has good visualization of that end point. Sometimes that means extending the incision higher on the internal carotid artery where it is very small. If that is the case, then it will be necessary to use the second method, which is to create a patch graft at the end of the procedure to enlarge the vessel. The patch can be made of several different materials which will be discussed later.

21. In which types of cases and under what circumstances do you feel a patch graft is necessary? What percentage of the cases that you treat require a patch graft?

A carotid patch can be used to make small carotid arteries larger, to change the flow characteristics near the end point of the carotid endarterectomy, and to decrease the thrombogenicity of the endarterectomized segment. Some surgeons patch all cases of carotid endarterectomy. Most surgeons patch some of them. The types of cases that are usually patched are those where the internal carotid artery is very small or where the patient has had a carotid re-stenosis requiring surgery a second time. Patches are also used where there is increased turbulence inside the vessel at the end of the procedure. When dealing with a marginal case, the surgeon should go ahead and patch. If the surgeon says he never patches, be wary.

22. If you patch, what type of patch do you use: (A) Dacron, (B) PTFE (Teflon), (C) autogenous vein graft, (D) bovine vein patch? Why do you prefer this type?

A patch angioplasty is a technique of placing a patch graft into the closure at the time of doing a carotid endarterectomy. Patches are most often used for small vessels, severely traumatized vessels, carotid re-stenosis requiring re-endarterectomy, and for vessels that have a lot of turbulence with thrill palpable through the wall of the artery at the end of the procedure. The purpose of the patch is to make the vessel larger, to improve the flow characteristics in the postoperative period, and to delay the atherosclerotic process.

Adding a patch to the procedure prolongs the operation fifteen to thirty minutes. Some type of monitoring to protect the brain from ischemia is necessary if one is patching, or else a shunt should be used during the procedure. Occasionally, there will be a delayed blowout of a saphenous vein patch because it was unable to withstand arterial pressure, but this is rare. It is also true that manufactured patches such as Dacron and PTFE slightly increase the risk of infection and false aneurysm formation, and they do not completely stop the reformation of plaque.

In general, patches are desirable overall and have some good benefits. Very careful attention must be paid to ensuring that the brain receives enough oxygen during the prolonged patch application time. In addition, if a saphenous vein patch is used, the vein should be from the proximal leg where the saphenous vein is stronger rather than from the region down around the ankle where the vein is weaker and may not be able to withstand arterial pressure. I think, as a patient, you may feel comfortable in the hands of a surgeon who shows some knowledge about patches and states that he uses them sometimes, or all the time, but probably it is wise to avoid using a surgeon who says that he never patches.

23. When you have completed an endarterectomy procedure and are ready to close the artery, do you start suturing from the top of the arteriotomy incision in the upper part of neck and sew down to the bifurcation to take advantage of the collateral circulation from the external carotid artery, or do you ignore this source of collateral circulation for the brain (see figure 4.2)?

When the common carotid artery is occluded, it is possible to allow blood from the branches of the external carotid artery to supply the brain for the remainder of the closure of the arteriotomy incision if the arteriotomy is closed in this manner. If a shunt is in place, this maneuver is less important, but for those non-shunted cases this is a wonderful source of collateral circulation which should be utilized.

24. Do you anticoagulate with heparin during the surgical procedure and continue to give some heparin during the first eight hours following the procedure?

Almost all vascular surgeons feel that any patient receiving an endarterectomy should be heparinized during clamp-off time. In addition, it has been shown that heparin during the first few hours following the completion of the operation helps to prevent thrombi from appearing in the recently endarterectomized segment. If the surgeon says that he does not feel heparin is necessary for this operation, it is probably best to ask the referring doctor to suggest a different surgeon.

25. Will I go to a recovery room after surgery?

Following a carotid endarterectomy it is vitally important for the patient to go to a recovery room where highly trained recovery room nurses are able to watch the patient every minute–monitoring the blood pressure, respiratory status, and cardiac rhythm, as well as the speech and neurological status of the patient. Most of the people who will have a serious complication from carotid endarterectomy will have that complication while still in the recovery room. If a neurological deficit develops in the recovery room, time is of the essence, and the surgeon must be notified immediately so that a decision can be made whether reoperation is necessary. Rarely, but occasionally, the endarterectomized portion of the carotid artery thromboses and emergency surgery is necessary to take out the thrombus and reestablish flow. Rapid response is extremely important in these cases. In addition, since the patients are often on heparin, a hematoma sometimes forms, which could cause respiratory distress if not recognized by a recovery room nurse and taken care of promptly by the surgeon. Occasionally, patients in the recovery room will have seizures which require immediate attention, or they may have bleeding or respiratory insufficiency. All of these things are usually correctable, and they are easier to correct if a recovery room nurse is nearby when they happen.

26. Will I go to an Intensive Care Unit after leaving the recovery room?

It is best to spend at least twelve hours in an Intensive Care Unit after leaving the recovery room to continue careful monitoring for high blood pressure, low blood pressure, neurological deficits, seizures, respiratory status, transient ischemic attacks, bleeding, and problems with speech or coordination. If any of these things occur, the surgeon will want to be notified immediately so that corrective action can be taken. In these days of cost-containment coverage, some articles have appeared in the literature saying that Intensive Care monitoring is not necessary following most carotid endarterectomies. I disagree with that opinion.

27. Will you pay special attention to making the incision in the neck in a small skin crease to reduce scarring?

It is wise for the surgeon to make the incision for endarterectomy in the direction of the lines of the skin so that the healing process will be prompt and nonpainful, and one will barely be able to see the final scar. If the surgeon does not pay special attention to that incision, a bad scar can appear on the neck, and wrinkling of the skin can occur.

28. Will you pay special attention to avoiding injury to the mandibular branch of the facial nerve so my lip will not sag postoperatively?

It is important for the surgeon to be aware that this nerve is in the region of the incision necessary for carotid endarterectomy. Careful attention to this fact will enable him to avoid injury. A sagging lip is the result of damage to the facial nerve, and often is permanent if it occurs. Unfortunately, it has happened in too many cases, and you will want to use a surgeon who is particularly mindful of the anatomy and the anatomic location of this nerve so that he can avoid injury to it. The marginal mandibular branch of the facial nerve is sometimes injured when the surgeon is making the initial incision for carotid endarterectomy. Harm can be avoided if the surgeon carefully curves the cephalic end of the incision posteriorly, aiming towards the mastoid process.

29. Will you pay special attention to avoiding injury to the hypoglossal nerve?

The hypoglossal nerve is close to the carotid bifurcation, and if this nerve is injured during the operative procedure the patient will lose some control and coordination of the tongue muscle. Swallowing will become more difficult, and the injury will be permanent. Make sure your surgeon will pay special attention to avoiding injury to this nerve. The hypoglossal nerve is one of the cranial nerves which is injured most frequently. It is located usually about 2 cm (slightly less than one inch) above the bifurcation of the carotid artery into its external and internal branches. It courses from lateral to medial, directly overlying the external carotid artery. If it is overstretched, bruised, or divided, the patient usually has unilateral tongue weakness, a lack of coordination with chewing, and less articulate speech. If the nerve is merely bruised and not divided, it will usually recover in several months. The surgeon can avoid injury by identifying the nerve early in the dissection process and avoiding traction in that area. Sometimes the nerve is stuck closely to the posterior aspect of the transverse facial vein. In this case, special care should be taken to avoid dividing the hypoglossal nerve when dividing the transverse facial vein.

30. Will you pay special attention to avoiding injury to the recurrent laryngeal nerve so I will not be hoarse after surgery?

The trunk of the vagus nerve travels in the carotid sheath posteriorly between the carotid artery and the jugular vein. It is sometimes in a different location, either anterior or lateral to the bifurcation of the carotid artery. Sometimes the vagus nerve curves itself over the carotid artery, right in the region the surgeon would like to make the arteriotomy incision. These cases require careful dissection in order to gain visibility without nerve damage. The superior laryngeal nerve descends posteriorly to the internal carotid artery until it reaches the level of the bifurcation, and then it divides. Sometimes placement of self-retaining retractors puts tension on this nerve as well as the recurrent laryngeal nerve. The trunk of the vagus nerve itself is sometimes injured by inadvertent inclusion with vascular clamps. Stretching, bruising, or dividing the superior laryngeal nerve causes high-pitched tones of the voice and easy fatigability of the voice. It also sometimes causes numbness at the base of the tongue and epiglottis, creating difficulty with swallowing and a predisposition to aspiration, particularly of liquids. If the recurrent laryngeal nerve is damaged, the patient will be hoarse postoperatively, sometimes for long periods of time and occasionally permanently. If the recurrent laryngeal nerve is injured, the patient develops paralysis of the unilateral vocal cord, and the patient has difficulty clearing secretions from his throat. The surgeon must be particularly careful when doing a carotid endarterectomy on the second side after a patient has previously developed injury to a recurrent laryngeal nerve on the first side, because bilateral paralyzed vocal cords can cause airway obstruction. The most common reason for hoarseness following carotid endarterectomy is not injury to the laryngeal nerve, however, but rather laryngeal edema, which usually subsides very rapidly. Keep this in mind if you should find yourself experiencing some postoperative hoarseness; it does *not* necessarily mean that there has been laryngeal nerve damage. In fact, even most patients with actual injury to the laryngeal nerves will regain nearly full function within six months, but the occasional case where the vocal cord paralysis lasts for an extended period of time can be treated successfully with Teflon injections on an out-patient basis.

The patient needs to understand that the surgeon cannot guarantee against injury to the laryngeal nerves, the hypoglossal nerve, the marginal mandibular branch of the facial nerve, or the vagus nerve. It is simply impossible to assure this with certainty in every case. Nonetheless, you want to be reassured that your surgeon is experienced in this type of procedure, knows which nerves to be especially alert for, and will make every effort to avoid injury.

31. What other possible complications can occur?

The surgeon will likely answer that during this operation one can have all of the usual complications of surgery, such as infection, hematoma, heart attack, and even death. The most common complication is stroke during the operation or within forty-eight hours. Those strokes are usually caused by small clots, emboli, or cerebral ischemia during the procedure and all of the technical factors which we have discussed above are designed to minimize the risk of these complications.

32. What is your personal risk of stroke during surgery or within forty-eight hours after the carotid endarterectomy procedure?

In the literature the risk is about 5 percent for symptomatic patients or 3 percent for asymptomatic patients, but you would like to know what this surgeon's personal success rate is. If the risk the surgeon gives you far exceeds the risks stated in the National Cooperative Studies, then perhaps you might want to consider a different surgeon.

33. Will you have a surgical assistant for the operation and have you used that surgical assistant on other carotid endarterectomy procedures?

A surgical assistant is an important part of the surgical team. A good assistant can make the operation run dramatically smoother and faster. If he uses a surgical assistant who has worked with him on many of these operations, the case will undoubtedly go smoother than if he has no assistant at all or is using a first-time assistant. The assistant could be another surgeon, a family practitioner who likes to assist and who has had a good deal of operating room experience, a nurse who is a trained RN first assistant, or a physician's assistant. All of these can make excellent surgical assistants for this procedure.

34. How soon should the operation be done?

It is never possible for a physician to predict exactly when a person will have a stroke from carotid stenosis, but some patients are having transient ischemic attacks, or they may have a critical stenosis as severe as 95 to 99 percent in a carotid artery; other special concerns would include a large, ulcerated plaque, or an ultrasound test which shows a thrombus moving around inside the lumen of the carotid bulb. In these instances, the operation should be done as soon as possible. Other cases can be scheduled in an elective fashion. You should listen to your surgeon concerning his recommendation for timing and try to have the operation done when he recommends that it be done.

35. Who will schedule the surgery?

Usually the surgeon's secretary will schedule the operation and write down for you the date you are to have the operation and the time you should report to the admitting office in the hospital. You must remember not to eat or drink anything for about twelve hours prior to going to the hospital because it will be dangerous for you to have an anesthetic if you have a stomach full of food or liquid. Some people get nauseated from the medication and start vomiting; they run the risk of sucking some of that fluid or food into their windpipe, causing aspiration pneumonia. Be sure to arrive at the hospital having not had anything to eat or drink recently.

36. Will I need additional testing to obtain medical clearance for surgery, and what preoperative lab tests will be necessary before the operation is done?

The most frequent nonsurgical complication of carotid endarterectomy is myocardial infarction, so it is likely that your physician will want to order a routine EKG and probably also a routine chest X-ray. If there is a history of significant lung disease, then you will also need to have arterial blood gas studies and pulmonary function tests performed. If heart disease is suspected, the operation should not be performed until after a cardiologist has evaluated the cardiac function. This will probably require an echocardiogram to measure the ejection fraction. If you have significant cardiovascular or pulmonary disease, it will be much safer for your operation to be performed under cervical block/local anesthesia, than with general anesthesia.[1]

37. When will the EEG wires be attached to my scalp, and will that hurt?

If your surgeon is using electroencephalographic monitoring during the procedure, the EEG wires will be attached to the scalp by the EEG technician, usually while you are in the holding area, about one hour before the operation. There is no real pain associated with the attachment of the EEG electrodes. Some technicians use collodion to help stabilize the electrodes to the scalp, and this must be cleaned from the hair postoperatively by the EEG technician.

38. What medications will I take after discharge?

The surgeon will probably allow you to resume all preoperative medications, and he may ask you to take aspirin or some other antiplatelet medication after discharge. In addition, if your cholesterol level is elevated you will probably be placed on a diet or medication to reduce the level. You must also stop smoking.

39. What will my activities be after surgery? When will I be allowed to be out of bed, when can I walk, and when can I drive a car and resume other activities?

The surgeon will probably allow you to be out of the bed into a chair by bedside about eight hours after surgery and will very likely allow you to walk to the bathroom with help within twelve hours after surgery. You should be able to drive a car within about seventy-two hours after surgery.

40. When will I be out of danger following the operation?

Most of the risk of stroke occurs during the operation and within twenty-four hours after the operation is completed. The good news is that if no stroke occurs during that period of time, it is unlikely that you will ever have a stroke from that carotid artery. Carotid re-stenosis does occur, but the re-stenosis rate is low and even that is correctable.

41. How often does carotid stenosis recur? Is it possible that I would need to have another carotid endarterectomy on that artery in the future?

It is possible for carotid stenosis to recur. It ordinarily takes many years for carotid stenosis to reach the dangerous stage after the first endarterectomy, but recurrent carotid stenosis does occur. After the atherosclerotic plaque is removed at the time of the first carotid endarterectomy, the atherosclerotic process begins again and new deposits of calcium and cholesterol start to form. In addition, there is sometimes mild intimal hyperplasia which builds up inside the artery, adding to the stenosis, so that it is possible, but unusual, for a significant re-stenosis to recur within one to two years. In general, however, the re-stenosis rate is about 1 percent per year, so that if one hundred carotid endarterectomies were done today, in ten years, ten of those people would have built up enough re-stenosis so that it would be necessary to perform the operation again. The re-stenosis is not as dangerous as the primary stenosis because it tends not to ulcerate as early or as severely as the primary carotid stenosis plaque. The re-stenosis can be primarily composed of new plaque, it can be primarily composed of hyperplasia of the intima, or it can be primarily scar formation. In any event, it is possible to correct the re-stenosis, but usually it is advisable to have a patch placed at the site of the re-endarterectomy to make the artery larger and to reduce the chances for a second re-stenosis. If one requires a re-endarterectomy with patch graft, the risk involved is slightly increased, but not much greater than the risk of the primary carotid endarterectomy. In my report of 7,854 carotid endarterectomies there were only two cases that required the same artery to be cleaned out three times, and both of those were patients who had diabetes mellitus.

42. What can be done to prevent the carotid stenosis from coming back?

In order to try to delay a recurrence of carotid stenosis it is important to stop smoking, avoid second-hand smoke, stay on a low cholesterol diet, and exercise regularly. It is also wise to have cholesterol testing to assure that your cholesterol level, HDL level, and LDL levels are within normal limits. Diabetic patients should stay under careful control. Even though you do all of these things, however, it is still possible to get a carotid re-stenosis. Prospective studies are being done to check the feasibility of using angioplasty with stent insertion for primary carotid stenosis and for carotid re-stenosis. The early results which have been reported indicate that angioplasty with stent insertion likely will not be a very safe procedure for primary carotid stenosis, but the preliminary results are favorable for angioplasty and stent insertion for carotid artery re-stenosis. The final results of the cooperative studies on these treatment options should be available in about two years.

43 Why can't I just take aspirin to prevent blood clots and not have the operation?

Aspirin with other anti-platelet aggregation agents are helpful in those patients with less that 60 percent stenosis and should be advised along with a recommendation to stop smoking, exercise daily, and eat a healthy diet. If the carotid stenosis is 60 to 90 percent, however, carotid endarterectomy is usually indicated. Aspirin helps to prevent thrombi, but in cases of more than 60 percent obstruction, aspirin alone is not adequate treatment.

44. Are you willing to take care of me after all of these questions?

Most surgeons will be delighted that you are informed about carotid endarterectomy. He or she will be glad that you asked the questions and will be happy to convince you of his awareness of all of these points. If, however, you are in the office of a surgeon who is offended by your questions and if he no longer wants to deal with you because of your having asked them, then it is just as well for you to be referred to another surgeon. It is unlikely that will be the case.

CHAPTER SIX

Anesthesia

General Anesthesia

Carotid endarterectomy can be done under general endotracheal anesthesia or under local cervical block anesthesia. The complications which can occur during or immediately following the operation include the risk of stroke and acute myocardial infarction and nerve injury to the hypoglossal nerve, recurrent laryngeal nerve, or facial nerve. The most common serious complication is stroke occurring during or immediately following the operative procedure. Such strokes are usually caused by emboli which develop during manipulation of the artery or particles of platelet thrombi which can appear on the raw surface of the internal wall of the artery after the endarterectomy procedure. Total occlusions can occur secondary to thrombi or intimal flaps. Intimal flaps can form as a result of clamps or tapes sometimes used with certain indwelling shunts during the operative procedure to protect the brain from ischemia during clamp-off time. Approximately 20 percent of patients develop ischemia when the carotid artery is clamped prior to opening the artery for removal of the plaque. If one uses general anesthesia without some type of monitoring procedure, it is not possible to determine which patients have ischemia and require an internal shunt and which do not. If a patient is having the operation done under general anesthesia, it is best for the surgeon to shunt every case. If a surgeon wishes to shunt only those patients who need one because of ischemia, then some type of monitoring is necessary. Methods of monitoring during the procedure include measurement of stump pressure, electroencephalogram, or transcranial Doppler. Those who prefer general anesthesia usually prefer it because they think it has better potential for controlling the airway and enables the anesthesiologist to use an anesthetic such as isoflurane, which slightly reduces the metabolic demand of the brain. In addition, the sleeping patient does not complain or remember the operative procedure. There is no discomfort even when high dissection is necessary. The operation can be done under a light general anesthetic with EEG monitoring in a safe and efficient manner. It is probably wise, however, to be more generous in selecting those patients who need shunting when general anesthesia is used. If general anesthesia is used without monitoring, then all patients should be shunted during the procedure.

Local Cervical Block Anesthesia

The carotid endarterectomy procedure also can be done under local cervical block anesthesia. In that case, the patient is given some mild IV sedation such as Versed, followed by injection in the side of the neck with local anesthesia agents such as Carbocaine or lidocaine. If the operation is to be performed under local anesthesia, then the patient can be neurologically monitored during the time of clamp-off of the carotid artery and a shunt is necessary only in those cases that develop some neurological changes. Local anesthesia has been used by some surgeons since the operation was first developed. If the patient is under local anesthesia, the surgeon can easily decide whether a shunt is needed or not. For additional safety, it is possible to monitor with EEG and also use local cervical block anesthesia. If the local anesthetic block is not completely satisfactory, however, some patients can have some discomfort requiring the anesthesiologist to give more sedation. In general, the blood pressure is less labile during local anesthesia than under general anesthesia.

I prefer the operation to be done under local or cervical block anesthesia and feel it is safer than general endotracheal anesthesia. I also feel that it is better to monitor with EEG in addition to using cervical block anesthesia and shunt only those patients who require it. This way the surgeon is always aware of the neurological status of the patient, and, if necessary, he can make changes to increase the blood supply to the brain. In the personal series of carotid endarterectomies I have performed, many patients had the operation done under general anesthesia for one side and the other side under cervical block anesthesia at a later time. The majority of those patients stated afterward that they preferred the cervical block anesthesia rather than the general anesthesia. There were fewer pulmonary complications and fewer problems with labile blood pressure and nausea. In addition, there was a low complication rate due to stroke or myocardial infarction.

In order to do a very good cervical block anesthesia, the anesthesiologist needs to perfect his technique. Once it is perfected, he is almost universally successful in getting a good block. A good block is essential for the patient to be comfortable during the operative procedure. I have worked with at least twenty different anesthesiologists who routinely performed excellent cervical block anesthesia for the operation, but a few anesthesiologists seem to have trouble mastering the technique. I have included here the technique for cervical block anesthesia which was used by one outstanding anesthesiologist who almost uniformly had a perfect result, meaning that the patient was able to undergo the operative procedure in an awake state without pain. He has allowed me to include his technique for that procedure in this book.[1]

For Physicians: Preferred Technique for Performing Cervical Block Procedure

For a patient undergoing cervical block for carotid endarterectomy surgery, two milligrams of midazolam (Versed) should be given intravenously preoperatively. Then 30 milligrams of ketorolac (Toradol) intravenously can be given if it is approved by the surgeon. The patient is then wheeled into the operating room and placed on the operating room table. Position is very important for this type of surgery. The patient's head should be almost at the far end of the table, nearly to the point where the head is falling off the table. This is done because the head of the table is cracked, and the junction of the table must be where the patient's neck is. The patient should also be close to the edge of the table on the side that is being operated on. One cc of fentanyl is then given intravenously, and the patient is placed in a Trendelenburg position. An inner scalene block is done with approximately 10 cc of 1.25 percent mepivacaine or Carbocaine with bicarb in 1 to 200,000 epinephrine. This solution is made with 1 and 1.5 percent mepivacaine (Carbocaine) mixture and put into three 20 cc syringes. Each 20 cc syringe will also contain 2 cc of bicarb, and 0.1 cc of epinephrine. This will result in a solution of 1.25 percent Carbocaine with 1 to 200,000 epinephrine with bicarb. Again, the inner scalene groove is palpated, a 20-gauge angiocatheter is placed in the groove, and 10 cc of the local anesthetic solution is placed with patient's head down and the anesthesiologist's fingers distal to the injection site to force the solution upward toward the cervical plexus. Next, the attention is turned to the deepest cervical plexus block, and the areas at C2, C3, C4, and C5 vertebrae are marked out. Also a line is made along the posterior border of the sternocleidomastoid muscle and along the carotid artery pulsation near the surgical site. The area is sterilely prepped, and the anesthesiologist uses a 10 cc syringe and a 22-gauge needle to inject at each vertebral level for the deep cervical plexus block. The tubercle is touched with the needle, and the attempt is made to fall into the trough of the tubercle where the nerve root is. As each tubercle is hit with the needle, approximately 3 to 4 cc of local anesthetic solution is injected there. Then, the superficial cervical plexus is injected along the posterior border of the sternocleidomastoid muscle with a skin infiltration. The superficial skin is infiltrated above the area of carotid pulsation. The mastoid process is infiltrated also. 1 cc of fentanyl can be given before all these injections. The patient is then placed in a reverse Trendelenburg position, the head-up position, and the head of the table cracked. During the surgery, another 2 to 4 milligrams of Versed can be given intravenously along with another 1 to 2 cc of fentanyl, making a total of 4 cc intravenously throughout the case. Phenylephrine (Neo Synephrine) should be drawn, and the patient's blood pressure should be maintained at least 140 to 160 mmHg for systolic blood pressure. During the clamp-off time, the anesthesiologist grasps the patient's hand and makes sure that the hand opposite the surgical area can be squeezed adequately by the patient. Pressure is maintained throughout in the 140 to 160 mmHg area. Oxygen is given by nasal cannula throughout the case, and an A-line can be started on the surgical or nonsurgical radial artery side. A Mayo stand can be brought in from the opposite surgical site. If needed during the surgery, midazolam (Versed) should be given in approximately 1/2 milligram aliquants. Heparin 10,000 milligrams is given intravenously, approximately five minutes before clamp-off time, and when the surgeon requests it 50 mg of Protamine is used at the end of the case. Hand squeezing commences when the surgeon clamps off the carotid artery, and ends when the patient's neck is starting to be closed. Close contact should be maintained with the EEG technician to let him know the patient is able to squeeze the hand, and also the EEG technician needs to know the blood pressure periodically. Assurance is given to the patient the whole time. Drapes are kept off the patient's face so he or she does not get a claustrophobic feeling. The surgical site arm is tucked to the side, and the opposite arm is out on an arm board.

CHAPTER SEVEN

Stroke Prevention Today

New Emergency Treatment for Acute Strokes

*I*f a person has a transient ischemic attack or develops any type or neurologic deficit, it is very important that he or she be taken to an emergency room as quickly as possible. There a physician can quickly evaluate and perform tests to determine if it is a TIA or if a stroke has recently occurred. A brain scan should be done immediately so that if there is an ischemic stroke rather than a hemorrhagic stroke the person could be considered for treatment with tissue plasminogen activator (t-PA). In order for the tissue plasminogen activator to work efficiently, it must be given within three hours of the onset of the symptoms of the stroke. If the patient arrives at the emergency room soon enough, and if the physician recognizes the symptoms and performs the testing rapidly enough, the t-PA can often dissolve the clot. This reestablishes blood supply to the brain, minimizing the damage or completely preventing the stroke. Each patient must be evaluated individually before a recommendation for t-PA is given because approximately six out of one hundred patients who receive the drug under these circumstances develop bleeding into the brain. A large cooperative study, however, found that under appropriate circumstances the benefits of t-PA substantially outweigh the risks. The National Institute of Neurological Diseases and Stroke has published a detailed protocol for selection of patients and method of treating patients with t-PA.

Only a neurologist or an emergency physician should make the decision for giving t-PA based on the patient's meeting certain specific criteria as far as age and as far as the time that the person presents for treatment. If the t-PA treatment is successful and the patient's neurological status returns to normal, then the patient will need a work-up to determine if carotid stenosis is present. If carotid stenosis is the underlying cause of the problem, the patient will need to have carotid endarterectomy in the near future for removal of the obstructing plaque in order to prevent additional strokes from occurring.

Surviving and Avoiding Stroke

Stroke is the third largest killer and approximately 730,000 people per year have a stroke in the United States alone. Stroke can be caused by a large list of conditions, but many physicians now agree that between 60 and 65 percent of strokes are caused by carotid stenosis. Atrial fibrillation with emboli to the brain causes 15 percent and hypertension with cerebral hemorrhage causes 10 percent. The thrombus frequently found in a middle cerebral artery of the brain actually formed in the carotid artery in the neck and is usually not a local thrombosis of the middle cerebral artery. This change in knowledge is extremely important because carotid stenosis in the neck can easily be diagnosed and treated to prevent a stroke.

Many of the patients who have a stroke do not die, but they do suffer serious long-term disabilities often requiring years of nursing home care. As we have seen, it is now possible to perform relatively simple screening tests to determine those patients who are at risk for these three major causes of stroke. I have offered specific guidelines here in an effort to help all of us understand what we can do to reduce the chances of stroke in ourselves and our loved ones. This book is a road map to help guide physicians and patients alike on a pathway toward more effective stroke treatment and prevention. In addition to the specific guidelines I have discussed at length, certain general principles remain important, including the change to a healthier lifestyle that will slow down the development of atherosclerotic plaques in your arteries. This lifestyle should include adequate exercise, a low cholesterol diet, and no smoking. You should find out whether or not you have diabetes mellitus and treat it if you do. If you have an irregular pulse, tests should be done to rule out atrial fibrillation, and if you have hypertension it should be treated. Make sure your serum cholesterol is below 200 and HDL and LDL and triglyceride fractions are normal. If diet alone does not result in a normal lipid profile, then medication should be taken to reduce the cholesterol and correct the abnormal HDL and LDL fractions and the triglycerides. It is important to do these things to slow down the atherosclerotic process. Recent research indicates that lowering the cholesterol levels protects against vascular disease. Make sure your primary physician listens to your neck arteries when you have an annual physical examination. By the time you reach age fifty, you should get screening tests for carotid stenosis, atrial fibrillation, and hypertension.

It is certainly important to help prevent or slow the development of plaque in our arteries by not smoking, getting adequate exercise, and making sure our serum cholesterol, triglyceride levels, and blood pressure are normal. However, these practices just help delay or prevent strokes for the long-term. If we want to be sure we are not at risk for having a stroke now or in the immediate future, we have to have our carotid arteries checked with an ultrasound test because partial obstruction in the carotid artery is the most important condition likely to cause a stroke. The ultrasound screening tests cost about $35 and are offered by several large screening companies and sometimes by local hospitals. By age fifty we should also be screened for atrial fibrillation and hypertension.

It is true that we have some exciting new methods for treating acute strokes, but it is much better to prevent strokes than to treat them after they have occurred.

Appendix

Inexpensive Screening for Stroke

An interview by Life Line Screening with
J. Crayton, Pruitt, M.D., P.A.
Diplomate of the American Board of Surgery
Diplomate of the Board of Thoracic Surgery

Since March 1997 1 have been the National Medical Director of Life Line Screening. In 1998, I was interviewed by its coordinator, Gina Johnson. Since our conversation reviews many of the important issues and questions regarding the benefits and procedures of screening for stroke, I have included the text here as an appendix.

1. What benefit do you see in a screening service for seniors?

A. Doctors are always interested in identifying people who are at risk for stroke. Fortunately, we have a very good tool for doing that: the ultrasound machine. It is quite accurate in being able to fairly inexpensively and noninvasively identify those people who are most at risk. We'd like everyone to know as much as possible about their health, including how likely it is for them to have a stroke. Many seniors have hypertension, diabetes, history of stroke, and high cholesterol. These things might increase their risk for stroke. Some have irregular heartbeat and are still smoking. It took many years to complete the National Cooperative Studies demonstrating that carotid endarterectomy was effective for prevention of stroke in asymptomatic people, and now that the information is available it is important to try to find those people who are asymptomatic so far but who have a significant carotid stenosis, since carotid stenosis probably causes as many as 60 to 65 percent of all strokes.

2. Don't you agree that it should be left up to the physician alone to determine when and what studies are indicated?

A. If a physician wants to do a complete ultrasound carotid test and the patient is completely asymptomatic, he or she is not really at liberty to order a complete test because it costs over $200. Medicare, Medicaid, and the insurance companies do not want us to order expensive tests like that on someone who is asymptomatic. However, if the individual would like to have himself tested to see if he is one of those asymptomatic people who has developed a significant stenosis, then for just $35 he can have this screening test. And if he ends up with a report that says he seems to have a moderate or severe stenosis, he may take that to his physician, and the doctor, armed with the results of tests, will feel comfortable ordering a complete carotid and vertebral test. Certainly, additional testing would be necessary before a definite diagnosis could be made or treatment recommended.

APPENDIX

3. **But an elderly patient (on a fixed income) who has been charged $35 for a screening test could then be charged $200 for a study that could have been initiated with her own physician.**

A. No, if a physician orders the test, then Medicare, Medicaid, and the insurance companies will pay for it. So the individual pays only the $35 for the initial screening test.

4. **Do you feel that seniors are being manipulated into taking these tests through a fear of stroke instilled by Life Line Screening?**

A. No, I think that the screening test allays fears because many of these people are already scared to death of having a stroke. Her husband has had a stroke, her sister has had a stroke; and her fears are allayed if she has the screening test and finds out that so far she herself has no stenosis or has only mild plaques.

5. **Isn't it true that some cases of "only mild stenosis" have led to stroke?**

A. Carotid stenosis does not cause all strokes. It probably causes about 60 to 65 percent of them. Some estimates are lower. Strokes may also come from hemorrhage into the brain or emboli from the heart or from ulcerated plaques in other arteries. But even if you accepted the lowest of the estimates, you would still be screening for the primary cause of strokes.

6. Does a screening test result of "only mild stenosis" instill a false sense of security in seniors?

A. Screening programs should be educational programs. Videos and pamphlets are presented which go into depth explaining the causes of stroke and how to prevent stroke. In addition to learning about carotid stenosis, seniors will find out that there are other things that they need to watch for, including hypertension, hypercholesterolmia, and irregular heart rhythm such as atrial fibrillation. The importance of stopping smoking is emphasized.

7. One of the controversies regarding a mass screening service such as this one is the issue of profiteering.

A. There does not appear to be a more economical, better method of discovering which asymptomatic people have significant carotid stenosis. I think it is amazing that Life Line is able to do high-tech screening for such an inexpensive price. They not only screen, but provide educational benefits as well.

The National Stroke Association also advocates and does screening and does a lot of teaching. The NSA carotid screening program, however, consists of listening with a stethoscope for bruits rather than performing an abbreviated duplex ultrasound test. The ultrasound is much more accurate and still relatively inexpensive. Individuals should learn how often they need to have a screening so they don't have the tests more often than necessary. Screening companies should be careful not to over-encourage the frequency of testing they recommend.

8. Then why don't physicians endorse what Life Line is doing?

A. I think that there are a great number of physicians who do understand the importance of screening for carotid stenosis, atrial fibrillation, and hypertension. Physicians are concerned because so many people are totally asymptomatic until a stroke occurs.

9. How can the public be assured that the methods and equipment utilized by Life Line Screening are good?

A. Life Line is using ultrasound machines which are of good quality and include color flow and Doppler. They use ultrasound technologists who are well qualified for doing this work. They have the same qualifications as ultrasound technologists in our hospitals. The test results, with suggestions for additional testing if needed, are sent to the individuals. Certified Letters are sent to those who appear to have a significant stenosis. I believe that screening is the most efficient and inexpensive way to find out if one has carotid stenosis.

10. Does Life Line Screening refer patients to you?

A. No. However, the physicians, upon receiving the report that their patients seemed to have a significant carotid stenosis, often have referred their patients to me for further diagnostic testing and possible surgical treatment of the disease. Many of these patients did require surgery, and I operated on them. They did have, in every instance, what the original Life Line ultrasound test had shown.

11. Some people feel that Life Line Screening endorses the carotid endarterectomy as a preferred form of treatment.

A. If a person has a 60 percent stenosis or greater, proven by ultrasound and by arteriography, then it has been established that the most effective method of preventing a stroke is by carotid endarterectomy. National Cooperative Studies showed that to be true. Most of the people being screened have less disease than that at the time of their screening and do not need to have surgery. Many, however, discover that plaques are developing in the carotid arteries. These people may have to reduce their blood cholesterol levels and control hypertension and stop smoking. Some may need to take aspirin or other antiplatelet medication. At some point, their physicians will need to decide if their patients are, in fact, stenotic enough to require surgery. Each individual who appears to have a significant stenosis should take the report to his or her physician and seek further advice or testing.

12. Why involve a screening service when the physician can identify a bruit and then refer the patient for proper evaluation?

A. If a person has a bruit, it may be significant. However, many patients who have even a 90 percent blockage with carotid stenosis have no bruit. Also, when we hear a bruit, we have no way of knowing if it is coming from the external carotid or the internal carotid. If it is coming from the external carotid, that blood supply is primary to the scalp and the face, and it is not necessarily significant. The internal carotid goes straight to the brain, and a bruit there is ordinarily significant. But the carotid duplex color Doppler ultrasound is much, much more accurate than listening with a stethoscope or listening with Doppler.

13. Some medical experts believe that it is best left up to the physician to determine when, where, and if ultrasound testing should be ordered. Do you agree?

A. If a doctor hears a bruit, then it is proper for him to order a complete carotid ultrasound test. Medicare, Medicaid, and most private insurance companies will pay for that. But if the patient has no bruit and is totally asymptomatic, then it is too expensive to allow every doctor to order a complete test. If an inexpensive ultrasound screening test suggests significant stenosis, however, the doctor can order a complete diagnostic ultrasound examination and Medicare and Medicaid and most insurance companies will pay for it.

14. Medical experts question the quality and accuracy of any ultrasound screening test performed for $35. What do you think?

A. The test is not considered to be adequate to make a definite diagnosis or to advise surgery: This is a screening test. It is, however, adequate to determine if the patient appears to have a significant blockage so that he needs to have additional testing in order that he might be encouraged to modify his lifestyle, take some medication, or have additional testing which might indicate a need for surgery.

15. Don't you feel that it is better for a patient to start the process with his or her physician as opposed to a screening service?

A. The person could start with a physician. But if that person is asymptomatic, then the doctor is going to be in the position of feeling that it is not completely legal for him or her to order a test on an asymptomatic patient just because that patient wants to have a test.

16. Do you question the legality of carotid screening services?

A. No, these programs can be beneficial and educational for the individual. The person determines if he wants to spend $35 to learn more about his carotid artery status. If he finds that he has a significant blockage, he may take the screening report to his doctor; then the physician would be quite comfortable ordering a complete test.

17 How accurate are these ultrasound tests?

A. Ultrasound is the most accurate test we have that is non-invasive and allows us to diagnose this condition. It is at least 95 percent accurate.

18. How is it possible to perform an ultrasound test in three to ten minutes?

A. The machines are quite expensive, the technologists are well-trained, and the programs for screening are well organized. The people understand the procedures they are going through. It is not a painful test; it is not a frightening test. So it is possible to accurately visualize the inside of these arteries—the common carotid, external carotid, and internal carotid artery—and measure the velocity of the blood going through those arteries in that length of time.

19. Some medical experts state that there is very little data to justify mass carotid vascular screenings. Do you agree?

A. There is no data that says it is not a good idea to screen people. The National Stroke Association recommends screening, as do many physicians. I know that some physicians do not employ ultrasound because it is a more expensive screening procedure than listening with a stethoscope. The stethoscope is helpful in finding bruits and for diagnosing atrial fibrillation, but it is not as accurate as carotid screening with color flow Doppler which can also measure velocity of the blood in the arteries. Several articles have been published documenting the accuracy and cost-effectiveness of carotid screening.

20. Are you being paid by Life Line for a professional endorsement?

A. No. Prior to the first of April 1997, 1 was only associated with Life Line through the fact that I was a busy vascular surgeon who did a lot of carotid endarterectomies. Some of those patients who had been found to have carotid stenosis learned about it at a Life Line screening and went to their physicians. The physicians then confirmed the findings of Life Line, that there was a significant stenosis, and then referred the patients to me for treatment. In April 1997, I was asked by Life Line to read some of their tests. I have been doing that for them, and I am paid for each test that I read.

21. Do you feel that you are biased in favor of carotid screening programs?

A. I think screening is great for educating people and finding carotid stenosis before the person who is asymptomatic has a stroke. If everyone who was going to have a stroke had a symptom first, we would probably not need screening. But since almost half of the people who suffer strokes have no symptoms beforehand, it is essential that we have a screening program. Carotid screening programs that utilize an abbreviated ultrasound test are particularly beneficial.

22. If you had a criticism of carotid screening organizations, what would it be?

A. I really think that these organizations do a remarkable job in trying to educate people without scaring them. It is amazing what they are able to do at such an inexpensive price.

23. You do not see a problem with the potential loss of quality from testing "en masse"?

A. I do not think so. In fact, I feel that quality may be enhanced. Everyone at Life Line is focused upon these screening programs. They are focused on educating people about the warning signals for stroke, explaining the nature of TIAs, and helping people to understand what is important in trying to prevent a stroke. The technologists are doing the test over and over again, and they have become quite efficient, quite well-trained at doing these tests. I think that quality is enhanced at a volume screening.

24. And who is making certain that quality standards are maintained at every screening?

A. The tests are first done by qualified technologists using a high quality color flow duplex ultrasound machine. And if that technologist thinks that something significant has been found, a second technologist comes and looks at it. Photographs are taken, velocities are measured, and the results are sent to a board certified physician who further interprets the test. A report is sent to the individual, who takes it to his or her doctor. And before any type of treatment is instituted, further testing is done to confirm the screening test.

25. Hospitals have mandatory protocols that are followed very carefully to make certain that people are not hurt or taken advantage of. There are no such regulations imposed on Life Line Screening.

A. Life Line has worked hard to maintain quality control. The technologists in the hospital who do this test have the same training as the technologists who are employed by Life Line. My feeling is that they are taking all the necessary precautions.

26. Do you feel that the cost-versus-benefit analysis should be considered and that insurance providers should reimburse the cost of screening?

A. I'm really not certain how to answer that question. With mammograms, for example, there has been quite a controversy for years about under what circumstances and how often mammography should be reimbursed. They finally settled that it should be reimbursed within certain parameters. And perhaps certain parameters can be identified for stroke screening to be reimbursed as well. Heart disease, cancer, and stroke are the three big killers. There are more people who are having strokes and becoming disabled and dying from them than women who are having cancer of the breast. Yet today, at last, we do reimburse for mammography screening. It seems clear to me that there is a place for stroke screening. There is no doubt in my mind that it saves lives and that it would be cost effective in the long run. But as far as reimbursement is concerned, that issue will no doubt be subject to debate for years to come. At the present time, screening companies do not bill Medicare, Medicaid, or insurance companies for carotid screening. The payment for the test is made by the individuals who desire to have the test performed. It is not proper for a screening company to bill an insurance company, Medicare, or Medicaid for these tests because they were not ordered by a physician.

Notes

Notes

Chapter One

1. National Stroke Association Home Page. www.stroke.org (1998).

2. *Be Stroke Smart.* National Stroke Association Newsletter 11, no. 2 (1994): 3.

3. The National Institutes of Health, report in the *Los Angeles Times*, 1 October 1994; W. S. Fields, V. Maslenikov, J. S. Meyer, R. D. Remington, and M. McDonald, "Joint Study of Extracranial Arterial Occlusion," *Journal of the American Medical Association* 211 (1970): 1993-2003; M. S. Fiandaca, M.D., and J. H. Wood, M.D., "Diagnostic Evaluation of Cerebral and Retinal Ischemia," *Neurosurgery: State of the Art Reviews* 4, no.1 (May, 1989): 1-22; R. W. Barnes, M.D., "Gentle on My Mind: The Epidemiology of Stroke," *The Journal of Vascular Technology* 22, no. 1 (1998): 37-41.

4. W. S. Fields, V. Maslenikov, J. S. Meyer, R. D. Remington, and M. McDonald, "Joint Study of Extracranial Arterial Occlusion," *Journal of the American Medical Association* 211 (1970): 1993-2003; North American Symptomatic Carotid Endarterectomy Trial Collaborators, "Beneficial Effect of Carotid Endarterectomy in Symptomatic Patients with High-grade Carotid Stenosis," *New England Journal of Medicine* 325 (1991): 445-53; Executive Committee for the Asymptomatic Carotid Arteriosclerotic Study, "Endarterectomy for Asymptomatic Carotid Artery Stenosis," *Journal of the American Medical Association* 273 (1995): 1421-28; R. W. Hobson, D. G. Weiss, W. S. Fields, J. Goldstone, W. S. Moore, J. B. Towne, C. B. Wright, and Veterans Affairs Cooperative Study Group, "Efficacy of Carotid En-

darterectomy for Asymptomatic Carotid Stenosis," *New England Journal of Medicine* 328 (1993): 221-27.

5. Atrial Fibrillation Investigators, "Risk Factors for Stroke and Efficacy of Antithrombotic Therapy in Atrial Fibrillation: Analysis of Pooled Data from Five Randomized Controlled Trials," *Archives of Internal Medicine* 154 (1994): 1449.

6. P. A. Wolf, R. D. Abbott, and W. B. Kannel, "Atrial Fibrillation as an Independent Risk Factor for Stroke: The Framingham Study," *Stroke* 22 (1991): 983-88.

7. Louis R. Caplan, Mark L. Dyken, and J. Donald Easton, *American Heart Association Family Guide to Stroke: Treatment, Recovery, and Prevention* (New York: Times Books, 1994) 25.

8. R. W. Barnes, M.D., "Gentle on My Mind: The Epidemiology of Stroke," *The Journal of Vascular Technology* 22, no. 1 (1998): 37-41.

9. Russell L. Cecil, M.D., and Robert F. Loeb, M.D., *Textbook of Medicine,* ninth edition (Philadelphia: W. B. Saunders Company, 1955).

Chapter Two

1. H. Chiari, "Uever das Verhalten des Teilungswinkels der Carotis communis bei der Endarteritis Chronica Deformis," *Verh. Disch, Ges. Pathology* 9 (1905): 326.

2. E. Moniz, "L'encephalographic arterielle, son importance dans la localization des tumeurs cerebrales," *Revue Neurologique* (1927) 72.

3. H. C. Johnson and A. E. Walker, "The Angiographic Diagnosis of Spontaneous Thrombosis of Internal and Common Carotid Arteries," *Journal of Neurosurgery* 8 (1951): 631.

4. C. M. Fisher, "Occlusion of the Internal Carotid Artery," *Archives of Neurology and Psychiatry* 65 (1951): 340-377.

5. M. E. Debaky, "Successful Carotid Endarterectomy for Cerebrovascular Insufficiency: Nineteen Year Follow-Up." *Journal of the American Medical Association* 233 (1975): 1083.

6. H. H. G. Eastcott, G. W. Pickering, and C. G. Rob, "Reconstruction of Internal Carotid Artery in a Patient with Intermittent Attacks of Hemiplegia," *Lancet* 2 (1954): 994.

7. W. S. Fields, V. Maslenikov, J. S. Meyer, et al., "Joint Study of Extracranial Arterial Occlusion: Progress Report of Prognosis Following Surgery or Nonsurgical Treatment for Transient Cerebral Ischemic Attacks and Cervical Carotid Artery Lesions," *Journal of the American Medical Association* 211 (1970): 1993-2003.

8. M. L. Dyken and R. Pokras, "The Performance of Endarterectomy for Disease of the Extracranial Arteries of the Head." *Stroke* 15 (1984): 968.

9. J. D. Easton and D. G. Sherman, "Stroke and Mortality Rate in Carotid Endarterectomy: 228 Consecutive Operations," *Stroke* 8 (1977): 565.

10. D. A. Shaw, G. S. Venables, N. E. F. Cartlige, et al., "Carotid Endarterectomy in Patients with Transient Cerebral Ischemia," *Journal of the Neurological Sciences* 64 (1984): 45-53.

11. The EC/IC Bypass Study Group, "Failure of Extracranial Intracranial Bypass to Reduce the Risk of Ischemic Stroke: Results of an International Randomized Trial," *New England Journal of Medicine* 313 (1985): 1191-1200.

12. J. D. Easton and J. L. Walterdink, "Carotid Endarterectomy: Trials and Tribulations," *Annals of Neurology* 35 (1994): 5-17.

13. North American Symptomatic Carotid Endarterectomy Trial Collborators, "Beneficial Effects of Carotid Endarterectomy in Symptomatic Patients with High-grade Carotid Stenosis," *New England Journal of Medicine* 325 (1991): 445-453.

14. European Carotid Surgery Trialists' Collaborative Group, MRC European Carotid Surgery Trial, "Interim Results for Symptomatic Patients with Severe (70-90 percent) or with Mild (0-29 percent) Carotid Stenosis," *Lancet* 337 (1991): 1235-43.

15. M. R. Mayberg, S. E. Wilson, F. Yatsu, et al., "Carotid Endarterectomy and Prevention of Cerebral Ischemia in Symptomatic Carotid Stenosis," *Journal of the American Medical Association* 266 (1991): 3289-94.

16. Asymptomatic Carotid Artery Stenosis (ACAS), "Endarterectomy for Asymptomatic Carotid Artery Stenosis," *Journal of the American Medical Association* 273 (1995): 18.

17. National Institute of Neurological Disorders and Stroke, "Carotid Endarterectomy for Patients with Asymptomatic Internal Carotid Artery Stenosis," *Pre-publication Clinical Advisory* 1994.

18. P. A. Wolf, R. D. Abbott, and W. B. Kannel, "Atrial Fibrillation as an Independent Risk Factor for Stroke: The Framingham Study," *Stroke* 22 (1991): 983-88.

19. Patient Outcomes Research Team, "Secondary and Tertiary Prevention of Stroke, " Agency for Healthcare and Policy Research publication no. 95-0091 (Sept. 1995).

20. R. S. Stafford and D. E. Singer, "National Patterns of Warfarin Use in Atrial Fibrillation," *Archives of Internal Medicine* 156 (1996): 2537-41.

21. European Atrial Fibrillation Trial Study Group, "Secondary Prevention in Non-rheumatic Atrial Fibrillation after Transient Ischemic Attack or Minor Stroke," *Lancet* 342 (1993): 1255-62.

22. W. B. Kannel, R. D. Abbott, D. D. Savage, and P. M. McNamara, "Epidemiologic Features of Chronic Atrial Fibrillation: The Framingham Study," *New England Journal of Medicine* 306 (1982): 1018-22.

23. Patient Outcomes Research Team, "Secondary and Tertiary Prevention of Stroke," Agency for Healthcare and Policy Research

publication no. 95-0091 (Sept. 1995); R. S. Stafford and D. E. Singer, "National Patterns of Warfarin Use in Atrial Fibrillation," *Archives of Internal Medicine* 156 (1996): 2537-41.

24. L. R. Caplan, M. L. Dyken, and J. D. Easton, *American Heart Association Family Guide to Stroke: Treatment, Recovery, and Prevention* (New York: Times Books, 1994) 25.

Chapter Three

1. Executive Committee for the Asymptomatic Carotid Arteriosclerotic Study, "Endarterectomy for Asymptomatic Carotid Artery Stenosis," *Journal of the American Medical Association* 273 (1995): 1421-28.

2. *Be Stroke Smart.* National Stroke Association Newsletter 11, no. 2 (1994): 3.

3. Johnson, Gina, *A Physician's Introduction to Life Line Screening* (Cleveland, Ohio: Life Line, 1998).

4. G. S. Lavenson, Jr., "Carotid Screening: Preparing for the Future," *Vascular Ultrasound Today* 2 (1997): 63-70.

Chapter Four

1. J. D. Easton and D. G. Sherman, "Stroke and Mortality Rate in Carotid Endarterectomy: 228 Consecutive Operations," *Stroke* 8 (1977): 565.

Chapter Five

1. J. Louveau, et al., "Carotid Endarterectomy Under Regional 'Conductive Anesthesia,'" *Annals of Surgery* 196 (1982): 59-64.

2. J. C. Pruitt, "1009 Consecutive Carotid Endarterectomies Using Local Anesthesia, EEG and Selective Shunting with the Pruitt-Inahara Carotid Shunt," *Contemporary Surgery* 23 (1982): 49-58.

3. J. C. Pruitt and R. E. Morales, "Carotid Endarterectomy: A Report of 7854 Procedures Using Local Anesthesia, EEG Monitoring, Occlusion Catheters, and the Pruitt-Inahara Carotid Shunt," *Surgical Technology International IV* 1995: 325-332.

Chapter Six

1. D. A. Hirschauer, "Procedure for Cervical Block Anesthesia," Personal interview (1994).

Works Cited

Asymptomatic Carotid Artery Stenosis (ACAS). "Endarterectomy for Asymptomatic Carotid Artery Stenosis Asymptomatic Carotid Atherosclerosis Study." *Journal of the American Medical Association* 273 (1995): 18.

Atrial Fibrillation Investigators, "Risk Factors for Stroke and Efficacy of Antithrombotic Therapy in Atrial Fibrillation: Analysis of Pooled Data from Five Randomized Controlled Trials." *Archives of Internal Medicine* 154 (1994): 1449.

Barnes, R. W., M.D. "Gentle on My Mind: The Epidemiology of Stroke." *The Journal of Vascular Technology* 22.1 (1998): 37-41.

Be Stroke Smart. National Stroke Association Newsletter 11.2 (1994): 3.

Caplan, Louis R., M. L. Dyken, and J. D. Easton. *American Heart Association Family Guide to Stroke: Treatment, Recovery, and Prevention.* New York: Times Books, 1994.

Cecil, Russell L., M.D., and Robert F. Loeb, M.D. *Textbook of Medicine*, 9th edition. Philadelphia: W. B. Saunders Company, 1955.

Chiari, H. "Uever das Verhalten des Teilungswinkels der

Carotis Communis bei der Endarteritis Chronica Deformis." *Verh. Disch, Ges. Pathology* 9 (1905):326.

Debaky, M. E. "Successful Carotid Endarterectomy for Cerebrovascular Insufficiency; Nineteen Year Follow-up." *Journal of the American Medical Association* 233 (1995): 1083.

Dorland's Illustrated Medical Dictionary. 24th edition. W. B. Saunders and Company: Philadelphia and London, 1968.

Dyken, M.L. and R. Pokras. "The Performance of Endarterectomy for Disease of the Extracranial Arteries of the Head." *Stroke* 15 (1984): 968.

EC/IC Bypass Study Group. "Failure of ExtracranialIntracranial Bypass to Reduce the Risk of Ischemic Stroke: Results of an International Randomized Trial." *New England Journal of Medicine* 313 (1985): 1191-1200.

Eastcott, H. H. G., G. W. Pickering, and C. G. Rob. "Reconstruction of Internal Carotid Artery in a Patient with Intermittent Attacks of Hemiplegia." *Lancet* 2 (1954): 994.

Easton, J. D. and J. L. Walterdink. "Carotid Endarterectomy: Trials and Tribulations." *Annals of Neurology.* 35 (1994): 5-17.

Easton, J. D. and D. G. Sherman. "Stroke and Mortality Rate in Carotid Endarterectomy: 228 Consecutive Operations." *Stroke* 8 (1977): 565.

European Atrial Fibrillation Trial Study Group. "Secondary Prevention in Non-rheumatic Atrial Fibrillation after Transient Ischemic Attack or Minor Stroke." *Lancet* 342 (1993): 1255-1262.

European Carotid Surgery Trialists' Collaborative Group,

MRC European Carotid Surgery Trial. "Interim Results for Symptomatic Patients with Severe (70-90 percent) or with Mild (0-29 percent) Carotid Stenosis." *Lancet* 337 (1991): 1235-43.

Executive Committee for the Asymptomatic Carotid Arteriosclerotic Study. "Endarterectomy for Asymptomatic Carotid Artery Stenosis." *Journal of the American Medical Association* 273 (1995): 1421-8.

Fiandaca, M. S., M.D., and J. H. Wood, M.D. "Diagnostic Evaluation of Cerebral and Retinal Ischemia." *Neurosurgery: State of the Art Reviews* 4.1 (May 1989): 1-22.

Fields, W. S., et al. "Joint Study of Extracranial Arterial Occlusion: Progress Report of Prognosis Following Surgery or Nonsurgical Treatment for Transient Cerebral Ischemic Attacks and Cervical Carotid Artery Lesions." *Journal of the American Medical Association* 211 (1970): 1973-2003.

Fisher, C. M. "Occlusion of the Internal Carotid Artery." *Archives of Neurology and Psychiatry.* 65 (1951): 340-77.

Hirschauer, D. A. "Procedure for Cervical Block Anesthesia." Personal interview, 1994.

Hobson, R. W., et al. and Veterans Affairs Cooperative Study Group. "Efficacy of Carotid Endarterectomy for Asymptomatic Carotid Stenosis." *New England Journal of Medicine* 328 (1993): 221-27.

Johnson, Gina. "A Physician's Introduction to Life Line Screening." Cleveland, Ohio: Life Line, 1998.

Johnson, H. C. and A. E. Walker. "The Angiographic Diagnosis of Spontaneous Thrombosis of Internal and Common Carotid Arteries." *Journal of Neurosurgery.* 8 (1951): 631.

Kannel, W. B., et al. "Epidemiologic Features of Chronic Atrial Fibrillation: the Framingham Study." *New England Journal of Medicine* 306 (1982): 1018-22.

Louveau, J., et al. "Carotid Endarterectomy Under Regional 'Conductive Anesthesia." *Annals of Surgery* 196 (1982): 59-64.

Lavenson, G. S., Jr."Carotid Screening: Preparing for the Future." *Vascular Ultrasound Today* 2 (1997): 63-70.

Mayberg, M. R., et al. "Carotid Endarterectomy and Prevention of Cerebral Ischemia in Symptomatic Carotid Stenosis." *Journal of the American Medical Association* 266 (1991): 3289-94A

Moniz, E. "L'encephalographic Arterielle, son Importance dans la Localization des Tumeurs Cerebrales." *Revue Neurologique* 2: (1927): 72.

National Institute of Neurological Disorders and Stroke. "Carotid Endarterectomy for Patients with Asymptomatic Internal Carotid Artery Stenosis." Pre-publication Clinical Advisory (1994).

National Stroke Association Home Page. www.stroke.org (1998).

North American Symptomatic Carotid Endarterectomy Trial-Collaborators. "Beneficial Effect of Carotid Endarterectomy in Symptomatic Patients with High-grade Carotid

Stenosis." *New England Journal of Medicine* 325 (1991): 445-53.

Patient Outcomes Research Team. "Secondary and Tertiary Prevention of Stroke." Agency for Healthcare and Policy Research publication no. 95-0091 (Sept. 1995).

Pruitt, J. C. "1009 Consecutive Carotid Endarterectomies Using Local Anesthesia, EEG and Selective Shunting with the Pruitt-Inahara Carotid Shunt." *Contemporary Surgery* 23 (1982): 49-58.

Pruitt, J. C. and R. E. Morales. "Carotid Endarterectomy: A Report of 7854 Procedures Using Local Anesthesia, EEG Monitoring, Occlusion Catheters, and the Pruitt-Inahara Carotid Shunt." *Surgical Technology International* IV (1995): 325-32.

Shaw, D. A., et al. "Carotid Endarterectomy in Patients with Transient Cerebral Ischemia." *Journal of the Neurological Sciences* 64 (1984): 45-53.

Stafford, R. S. and D. E. Singer. "National Patterns of Warfarin Use in Atrial Fibrillation." *Archives of Internal Medicine* 156 (1996): 2537-41.

The National Institutes of Health, report in the *Los Angeles Times*, 1 October (1994).

Wolf, P. A., R. D. Abbot, and W. B. Kannel. "Atrial Fibrillation as an Independent Risk Factor for Stroke: The Framingham Study." *Stroke* 22 (1991): 983-88.

Suggestions for Further Reading

Listed below are some other books which have been written on this subject:

Ancowitz, Arthur, M.D. *The Stroke Book: One on One Advice about Stroke Prevention, Management, & Rehabilitation.* New York: William Morrow and Company, 1993.

Caplan, Louis R., M.D. *American Heart Association Family Guide to Stroke: Treatment, Recovery, and Prevention.* New York: Times Books, 1994.

Greenhalgh, R. M., M.D., and L. H. Hollier, M.D., et al., eds. *Surgery for Stroke.* London: W. B. Saunders, 1993.

National Institute of Neurological Disorders and Stroke. National Institutes of Health Publication No. 99222. Bethesda, Md. 1999.

Semple, Peter F. *An Atlas of Stroke.* New York: Parthenon Publishing, 1998.

Shimberg, Elaine F. *Strokes: What Families Should Know.* New York: Ballantine Books, 1990.

Wood, James H., M.D., et al., "Carotid Artery Surgery and Stroke." *Neurosurgery State of the Art Reviews* 4.1 (May 1989).

Other Useful Resources

Information

American Heart Association
7320 Greenville Avenue
Dallas, TX 75231
214-748-7212
http://www.americanheart.org

American Occupational Therapy Association
1383 Piccard Drive
P. O. Box 1725
Rockville, MD 20850-4375
301-948-9626

American Physical Therapy Association
1111 North Fairfax Street
Alexandria, VA 22314
1-800-999-2782

Dr. C. Everett Koop's Web Site
Health information from former U.S. Surgeon General
http://www.drkoop.com

Life Line Screening of America
9545 Midwest Avenue – Suite D
Cleveland, OH 44125
1-216-581-6556

National Stroke Association
1420 Ogden Street
Denver, CO   80218
http://www.stroke.org
1-800-STROKES   (1-800-787-6537)

U.S. Government Printing Office
Superintendent of Documents
Washington, DC   20402
202 783 3238
http://www.usgovernment.org

Equipment

The Pruitt-Inahara shunt and the Inahara-Pruitt shunt as well as the carotid endarterectomy dissector kit and the Pruitt Occlusion Catheter can be obtained from:

Horizon Medical Products (HMP)
One Horizon Way
Post Office Box 627
Manchester, GA 31816
1-800-472-5221
www.hmpvascular.com

Glossary

acute: Severe; of short duration, as opposed to chronic.

anastomosis: The surgical or pathological connection of two tubular structures.

aneurysm: A ballooning out of the wall of an artery or of the heart due to weakening of the wall by disease, injury, or an abnormality present at birth.

angiography: A diagnostic procedure in which a dye is injected into blood vessels that are then photographed using X-rays. Angiography is used to visualize the condition of arteries and veins and to confirm the presence of blood clots or other abnormalities.

anticoagulant: An agent that prevents blood from clotting.

aphasia: Difficulty speaking, understanding, writing, or reading caused by damage to the brain.

arrhythmia: An abnormal heart rhythm.

arteriography: A method of X-ray viewing the inside of the arteries by injection of radiopaque contrast substances into the lumen of the arteries.

arteriovenous malformation: A congenital condition in which arteries directly connect with veins instead of going through capillaries. Arteriovenous malformations are frequently associated with subarachnoid hemorrhage.

arteritis: Inflammation of an artery.

artery: A blood vessel that carries blood from the heart to the various parts of the body.

atherosclerosis: A type of artery disease in which the inner layers of artery walls become thick and irregular because of deposits of cholesterol and calcium. As the interior walls of arteries become thickened with layers of these deposits, the arteries become narrowed and the flow of blood through them is reduced. A localized area of this build-up is called an "atheromatous plaque" and is often referred to as "hardening of the arteries."

atrial fibrillation: The uncoordinated contractions of individual heart muscle fibers in the upper chambers of the heart. These chambers, called the atria, cannot contract in an organized fashion, and they pump blood ineffectively, if at all.

bifurcation: A separation into two branches; the point of forking.

blood clot: A mass of thickened blood formed by clotting factors in the blood. This clot can stop the flow of blood from an injury. Blood clots can form inside an artery whose walls are damaged by atherosclerotic plaques and can cause a heart attack or stroke. A blood clot and a thrombosis are the same.

brain hemorrhage: An uncontrolled bleeding in or on the brain.

bruits: Abnormal sounds or murmurs caused by turbulence and heard over blood vessels.

cardiac: Pertaining to the heart.

cardiovascular disease: Disease of the heart and blood vessels, including stroke, rheumatic heart disease, and high blood pressure.

cardioversion: An elective procedure in which a synchronized shock of 25 to 50 joules (watt seconds) is triggered by use of a defibrillator in order to restore the heart to normal sinus rhythm.

carotid artery: The major artery in the neck carrying blood to the brain. The body has a left carotid artery and a right carotid artery.

carotid endarterectomy: Surgical removal of atherosclerotic plaque deposits from the carotid arteries.

caudad: Toward the tail, posteriorly.

cephalad: Toward the head, anteriorly.

cerebral embolism: A blood clot formed in one part of the body and then carried by the blood stream to the brain where it lodges in an artery.

cerebral hemorrhage: Bleeding within the brain resulting from a ruptured blood vessel, usually caused by aneurysm, a head injury, or hypertension.

cerebral thrombosis: Formation of a clot in an artery that supplies blood to part of the brain.

cerebrovascular occlusion: The obstruction or closing of a blood vessel in the brain.

cholesterol: A type of fatty substance found in animal tissue. Cholesterol is present only in foods from animal sources, such as dairy products, meat, fish, poultry, animal fats, and egg yolks.

chronic: Having a long duration, as opposed to acute.

coarctation: Compression of the walls of a vessel or stricture of a vessel.

collateral blood flow: A system of smaller arteries, closed under normal circumstances, that may open up and start to carry blood around an obstructed artery.

computer tomography: A radiographic diagnostic test often used for evaluating brain tissue and identifying whether a

Glossary

stroke was due to bleeding or a blockage in an artery. Also called a CT scan or CAT scan.

congenital: Any condition present in the body at birth.

congestive heart failure: The inability of the heart to pump out all of the blood that returns to it. This results in blood backing up in the veins that lead to the heart and sometimes fluid accumulates in various parts of the body.

deficit: A term for a physical or cognitive disability.

diabetes mellitus: A disease in which the body does not produce or properly use insulin. Diabetes increases the risk of developing cardiovascular disease.

diastolic blood pressure: The lowest blood pressure measurement in the arteries. It occurs when the heart muscle is relaxed between beats.

dysphagia: Difficulty in swallowing or the inability to swallow, sometimes caused by brain damage or injury to hypoglossal nerve in the neck.

edema: Swelling due to an abnormally large amount of fluid in body tissue.

electrocardiogram: A graphic record of electrical impulses produced by the heart.

embolic stroke: A stroke caused by obstruction in a brain artery caused by a clot that has formed elsewhere, usually in the heart or in the carotid arteries, and has been carried through the blood stream to the brain.

embolus: A blood clot that forms in a blood vessel in one part of the body and then is carried to another part of the body. The pleural of embolus is emboli.

heart attack: Death of, or damage to, part of the heart muscle due to an insufficient blood supply. Also known as myocardial infarction.

hematoma: A tissue swelling filled with blood.

hemianopia: A partial blindness caused by damage to the brain. The vision is "blacked out" in the left or right visual field of both eyes.

hemiplegia: A paralysis of one side of the body.

hemorrhage: Profuse bleeding from a ruptured blood vessel.

heparin: A type of anticoagulant drug that prevents clotting by affecting the blood component fibrinogen.

high blood pressure: A chronic blood disease in which blood pressure is above its normal range of 140/90. High blood pressure increases the risk of heart disease and kidney disease and is a major risk factor for stroke. A technical term for high blood pressure is hypertension.

GLOSSARY

high density lipoprotein: A carrier of cholesterol believed to transport cholesterol away from the tissues and to the liver, where it can be excreted. Also called HDL. Sometimes called the "good cholesterol" in comparison to low density lipoprotein (LDL).

hyperlipidemia: An abnormally high concentration of lipids (fatty material) in the blood.

hypertension: Same as high blood pressure.

hyperplasia: The abnormal increase in the number of cells in a tissue causing increased thickness.

hypoperfusion: The inability of the vascular system to supply an outlying arterial area with blood, commonly due to a lack of blood pressure or an arterial blockage.

infarction: Death of tissue due to a lack of blood, usually caused by a blockage of an associated artery.

intermittent claudication: A complex of symptoms characterized by absence of pain in a limb when at rest. The start of pain and weakness when walking is begun, intensification of the pain and weakness if exercise is continued, and the disappearance of symptoms after a brief period of rest.

intima: The innermost layer of the wall or lining of a blood vessel.

intracerebral hemorrhage: Bleeding from an artery deep within the brain, causing pressure on the brain tissue.

ischemia: Decreased blood flow to an organ, usually due to constriction or obstruction of an artery.

lacunes: Small cavities in the substance of the brain. The cavities are believed to be caused by the death of tissue during a transient ischemic attack or mini stroke.

ligate: To tie or bind a blood vessel.

lipid: A fatty substance insoluble in blood.

lipoprotein: The combination of lipid surrounded by protein; the protein makes it soluble in blood.

low density lipoprotein: The main carrier of harmful cholesterol in the blood. Also called LDL and referred to as the "bad cholesterol" in comparison to high-density lipoprotein (HDL).

lumen: The inner part of a tube such as blood vessel.

magnetic resonance imaging: a noninvasive diagnostic tool which produces a magnetic field for examining the brain and other parts of the body. Also called MRI.

middle cerebral artery: A major artery of the brain which supplies most of the upper brain. Each cerebral hemisphere is supplied by a middle cerebral artery. Also called MCA.

myocardial infarction: The damaging or death of an area of the heart muscle resulting from a reduced blood supply to that area. A myocardial infarction is a heart attack.

neurologist: A physician who specializes in diagnosing and treating diseases of the brain and other parts of the nervous system.

occlusion: An obstruction of an artery by something such as a blood clot or thrombus.

P Waves: The electrical impulse of atrial contraction.

perfusion: The passage of a fluid (usually blood) through the vessels of an organ or body part.

peripheral nervous system: A collection of nerves that fan outward from the spinal column to reach every part of the body.

plaque: A deposit of fatty substances and calcium in the inner lining of the arterial wall.

platelet antiaggregant/platelet inhibitor: A class of drugs that prevent platelets from sticking together to form a blood clot. Aspirin and ticlopidine are examples of platelet antiaggregants.

platelets: One of the three kinds of formed elements found in the blood. Platelets aid in the clotting of the blood.

polyunsaturated fats: Oils of vegetable origin such as corn, safflower, sunflower, and soybean oils that are liquid at room temperature.

primary risk factor: Factor that directly affects the risk of stroke. Primary risk factors for stroke are high blood pressure, heart disease, cigarette smoking, previous stroke, age, sex, race, diabetes mellitus, and transient ischemic attacks.

R-R Interval: The elapsed time between two consecutive ventricular contractions.

resection: Partial excision of a bone or other structure.

rheumatic heart disease: Damage to the heart valves by inflammation caused by attacks of rheumatic fever.

risk factor: A condition which increases the chance of developing cardiovascular disease or stroke.

saturated fat: Type of fat found in foods of animal origin and occasionally of vegetable origin which are typically solid at room temperature.

secondary risk factor: Risk factors that indirectly affect the risk of stroke, by increasing the risk of heart disease or other primary risk factors. Obesity, high blood cholesterol levels, and excessive alcohol drinking are secondary risk factors for stroke.

stenosis: Narrowing or constriction of an opening or lumen, such as a blood vessel.

stent: A device used to hold a vessel open by providing support.

stroke: The sudden interruption of the blood supply to the brain, caused either by blockage or a rupture of blood vessels.

subarachnoid hemorrhage: Uncontrolled bleeding on the surface of the brain in the area between the brain and the skull.

systolic blood pressure: the highest blood pressure measured in the arteries. It occurs when the heart contracts with each heart beat.

thrombolysis: The breaking up of a blood thrombus or clot.

thrombolytic agents: Drugs that work by dissolving blood clots in arteries or veins.

thrombotic stroke: A stroke caused by a blood clot or thrombus that forms in an artery going to the brain. The clot blocks the passage of blood to a part of the brain.

thrombus: A blood clot that forms inside a blood vessel or cavity of the heart.

tissue plasminogen activator: A natural protein that works by dissolving blood clots in arteries, restoring blood flow inside of the artery. Also called t-pa. It is used for heart patients and for some stroke patients.

transcranial Doppler ultrasound: A noninvasive diagnostic test that uses ultrasound techniques to generate information about intracranial blood vessels. Also called TCD.

transient ischemic attack: An abnormal neurologic episode that is caused by a temporarily blocked blood vessel and leaves no permanent brain damage. Symptoms are the same as for a stroke, but are temporary, usually lasting twenty-four hours or less. They are an important warning sign of an impending stroke and should never be ignored. Also called TIA.

triglyceride: A fatty substance or lipid circulating in the blood.

ultrasound: Fast-frequency sound vibrations, not audible to the human ear, used in medical diagnosis.

vascular: Pertaining to blood vessels.

vasoconstriction: A narrowing in a blood vessel reducing the area through which blood may pass.

vein: Any one of a series of blood vessels of the vascular system that carries blood from various parts of the body back to the heart.

vertebral artery: One of two arteries in the back of the neck that supply the posterior part of the brain with blood.

warfarin: A synthetic anticoagulant that works by preventing certain blood clotting agents from forming in the liver.

Index

Index

A

abbreviated color flow duplex ultrasound. *See* ultrasound
activity after surgery, 98
adrenal tumors, 43
African Americans, 37
age, 13, 19, 65*fig*
amaurosis fugax, 30–31
anesthesia, 49–50, 69, 101–6
    cardiovascular disease, 96–97
    local vs. general, 103
    monitoring, 69–76
    pulmonary disease, 96–97
    sedation, 52, 69, 72, 102–6
    technique for cervical block, 104–6
    See also general anesthesia; local anesthesia
anesthesiologist, 54
aneurysm, 27–28
angina pectoris, 22
angioplasty with stent insertion, 100
anticoagulation, 22–23, 25, 40, 43, 89
    See also heparin
aphasia, 34
Argyle Shunt, 82*fig*
arm coordination, 19, 33, 64*fig*
arrhythmia. *See* cardiac arrhythmia
arterial blood gas studies, 96–97
arterial clamp positions, 53*fig*, 54
arteritis, 29
aspiration, 96
aspirin, 97, 100

asymptomatic atrial fibrillation, 23–25
Asymptomatic Carotid Atherosclerosis Study (ACAS), 14, 36
asymptomatic carotid stenosis, 4–6,
    14, 15, 17, 35–40, 64–65*figs*, 112
atherosclerosis, 2, 9, 17
  gender, 17
  hypertension, 41
  lifestyle, 99, 109
  patch grafts, 88
  recurrence of carotid stenosis, 98–99
  See also coronary artery disease
atrial fibrillation, 3, 24*fig*, 38, 108–9
  causes, 21–22
  diagnosis, 23–25, 42–43
  hypertension, 22
  incidence, 36
  screening tests, 40
  symptoms, 25
  treatment, 22–23
auricular fibrillation, 7, 39
autogenous vein grafts, 88

B

back-bleeding, 52, 54–55, 70
balloons, 79–84
  vs. clamps, 82–84
  occlusion catheters, 52, 54–56,
    62, 83–87, 84*fig*
  shunts, 62
bifurcation of the carotid artery, 9–10, 17, 29
  curved dissector, 60
  hypoglossal nerve, 92
  vagus nerve, 93–94
blood pressure, 74–76, 90
  local vs. general anesthesia, 103

monitoring, 61, 71, 106
normal, 27, 38
side ports, 79, 81
See also hypertension
bovine vein grafts, 88
brain blood supply, 17, 72–73
brain hemorrhage, 1, 3, 15, 27–28, 107
brain monitoring during surgery, 47–52, 54, 62–63, 69–76, 101–2, 106
brain scans, 15, 32, 47, 107
Brener Shunt, 78*fig*
bruits, 35, 38, 64–65*figs*, 116–17, 119

C

calcium deposits, 2, 17, 64–65*figs*
Carbocaine, 102, 104–6
cardiac arrest, 71
cardiac arrhythmia, 74–76
  during surgery, 61, 71
  side ports, 79
cardiac emboli, 26
cardiac status, 90
cardiology examination, 96–97
cardiovascular surgeons, 67–68
cardioversion, 22–23, 40, 43
carotid arteries, 16*fig*, 17, 42, 74
carotid artery bifurcation, 9–10, 17, 29
  curved dissector, 60
  hypoglossal nerve, 92
  vagus nerve, 93–94
Carotid Artery Risk Factor Ultrasound Study, 39–40
carotid bruits, 35, 38, 116–17, 119
carotid endarterectomy, 2–3, 10–12
  anesthesia, 49–50, 69, 101–6
  cerebral ischemia, 47, 51–52, 55, 75–76, 94–95

complications, 101–2
decision making process, 47, 100
vs. medical management, 3, 36, 48
morbidity and mortality, 11–12, 49*fig*
questions, 67–100
risks, 61–62, 91–98, 103
shunts, 51–52, 57, 62, 69–86, 77–82*figs*, 103
surgical procedures, 48–63, 101–4
carotid endarterectomy dissector kit, 59*fig*
carotid stenosis, 2, 10–11, 13, 18*fig*, 108
   age, 29–30
   angioplasty with stent insertion, 100
   asymptomatic, 4–6, 14, 15, 17, 35–40, 112
   diagnosis, 15, 31–42
   etiology of strokes, 17–20
   gender, 29–30
   incidence, 14, 36
   recurrence, 86, 88, 98–99, 100
   screening, 35–40, 109–10, 111–22
   surgery, 45–65, 95–96, 101–6
   ulcerated plaques, 29–30, 64–65*figs*
carotid ultrasound. *See* ultrasound
central retinal artery, 31
cerebral arteriography, 2, 9
cerebral ischemia, 47, 49, 51–52, 55, 71, 75–76, 94–95, 107
cerebral perfusion, 17, 72–73
cerebrovascular accident. *See* stroke
cervical block anesthesia, 49, 102–6
   See also local anesthesia
chest pain, 22
chest X-rays, 96–97
Chiari, H., 9
cholesterol, 17, 38, 39, 64*fig*, 97, 99, 109, 112
   See also hyperlipidemia
circulation. *See* collateral circulation

INDEX

clamp-off time, 72–73
   shunts, 69–70
clamps, 54, 57, 61–62
   vs. balloons, 82–84
classification of stroke, 7–8
clots, 3, 7
coarctation of the aorta, 43
collateral circulation, 53*fig*, 54, 56, 62, 70–71
   suturing, 89
complications, 101–2
   See also morbidity and mortality; risks
congestive heart failure, 13, 21–22, 42
coordination, 19, 33, 64*fig*
coronary artery disease, 21–22, 42
costs, 26, 117
   -benefit analysis, 121–22
Coumadin. *See* warfarin
cranial nerves, 53, 91–94, 101–2
CT scans. *See* brain scans
curved dissector, 59*fig*, 60
CVA. *See* stroke

D

Dacron patch grafts, 88
DeBakey, Michael, 10
diabetes, 13, 20, 99, 109, 112
diagnostic process, 29–43
   atrial fibrillation, 23–25, 42–43
   carotid stenosis, 4–5, 15, 31– 42, 116–17, 119
   hypertension, 43
   screening tests, 35–41, 111–22
disabilities due to stroke, 91–94, 109
dissectors, 58–62, 59*fig*
dizziness, 34
Doppler tests, 57, 70–72, *See also* ultrasound

double-blind studies, xviii. *See also* research
duplex carotid ultrasound, 32
dysarthria, 33, 92
dysphagia, 92–94

E

Eastcott, H.H.G., xvii, 10
Easton, J.D., 11
echocardiograms, 23, 43
educational programs, 114
EKGs. *See* electrocardiograms
electrocardiograms (EKGs), 23–25, 24*fig*, 40, 43, 96–97
electroencephalograms (EEGs), 72–74, 103
   monitoring, 49–52, 70–73, 102, 106
   procedure, 70–71, 97
elevators. *See* dissectors
emboli, 2, 17–19, 94–95, 101–2
   cardiac origin, 26
embolic strokes, 7–8, 18*fig*
emergency treatment, 107–8
endotracheal anesthesia. *See* general anesthesia
end points, 56, 62, 85–87
end-to-end anastomosis, 10
etiology
   atrial fibrillation, 21–26
   brain hemorrhage, 27–28
   carotid stenosis, 17–20
   historical views, 1–2
   statistics, 28
European Carotid Surgery Trial (ECST), 13–14
exercise, 99, 109
external carotid artery. *See* carotid arteries

F

facial nerve, 52, 91–92, 101–2

INDEX

fainting, 34
family history, 19
fasting, 96
father of author, xvii, 6–7
fear of stroke, 113
fentanyl, 104–6
fibromuscular hyperplasia, 29
Fisher, Miller, 9–10
flushing through side ports, 81
Freer elevator, 59*fig*

G

gender, 13, 17, 19
general anesthesia, 49–50, 75–76, 101–2
   cardiovascular disease, 96–97
   vs. local, 103
   monitoring, 69–76
   pulmonary disease, 96–97
grafts. *See* patch grafts

H

hand coordination, 33
hardening of the arteries. *See* atherosclerosis
headache, 34
heart attack. *See* myocardial infarction
heart valve prosthetics, 26
hematomas, 90
hemorrhage. *See* brain hemorrhage
heparin, 58, 62, 89, 106
high blood pressure. *See* hypertension
historical perspective, 1–2, 7, 9–12
hoarseness, 93–94
hospital choice, 68–69
hyperlipidemia, 13, 20
hypertension, 3, 13, 20, 41, 108, 109, 112

atrial fibrillation, 22
  brain hemorrhage, 27–28
  diagnostic process, 43
  screening, 39–41
hypoglossal nerve, 53, 92, 101–2

I

Inahara-Pruitt Shunt, 80*figs*
incidence of stroke, 1, 12–14, 36, 95, 108
  cardiogenic emboli, 26
incisions, 52, 62, 86–87
  plaque removal, 83
  vagus nerve, 93–94
insulin, 20
insurance coverage, 112–13
Intensive Care Units, 90–91
intermittent claudication, 13, 20
internal carotid artery, 17
  occlusion catheters, 83–87, 84*fig*
  shunts, 55
  See also carotid artery
internal jugular vein, 52
International Normalized Ratio, 25–26
intimal flaps, 56–58, 101–2
intimal hyperplasia, 98–99
intimal injuries, 82–85
intra-arterial digital carotid arteriogram, 42, 47
intravenous digital carotid arteriogram, 42
irregular pulse, 38
ischemia during surgery. *See* cerebral ischemia
ischemic strokes, 7–8, 11, 107
isoflurane, 102

J

Javid Shunt, 78*fig*

Johnson, H.C., 9
Joint Study of Extracranial Arterial Occlusion, 10–12

K

ketorolac (Toradol), 104
kidney disease, 43

L

Lancet (journal), 10
language changes, 34
laryngeal edema, 93–94
Lavenson, George S., Jr., 39–40
leg coordination, 33
leg pain, 13, 20
lidocaine, 102
Life Line Screening, 39, 111–22
lifestyle and atherosclerosis, 99, 109
limb function, 13, 19–20, 33, 64*fig*
limb numbness, 33
lip weakness, 91–92
local anesthesia, 49, 50–52, 69, 102–6
   cardiovascular disease, 96–97
   vs. general, 103
   monitoring, 69–76
   procedure, 72, 104–6
   pulmonary disease, 96–97
Loftus Shunt, 81*fig*
lone atrial fibrillation, 21
Longevity, Inc., 39
loss of consciousness, 73–74
lung disease, 96–97

M

Magnetic Resonance Angiogram (MRA), 42, 47
mandible, 52

manipulation of vessels, 61
Mayo Clinic, 51
Medicaid, 112–13
medical treatment
   atrial fibrillation, 3
   carotid stenosis, 3, 48
   hypertension, 3
   ischemic strokes, 107–8
   vs. surgical, 3, 36, 48
Medicare, 5, 112–13
medication, 97. *See also* anticoagulation
mepivacaine. *See* Carbocaine
midazolam. *See* Versed
middle cerebral artery, 7, 9–10, 108
monitoring during surgery, 47–52, 54, 69–76, 101–3, 106
monitoring, post-operative, 62–63
Moniz, E., 9
morbidity and mortality, 11–12, 48, 49*fig*
   surgeons, 15, 49*fig*
MRIs. *See* brain scans
myocardial infarction, 13, 20, 26, 103
   risks, 96–97, 101–2

N

National and International Cooperative Prospective Studies, 12–14, 112, 116
National Institute of Neurological Disease and Stroke, 14, 108
National Stroke Association, 114
   screening program, 37–38, 119
natural thyroid shunt, 53*fig*, 57
nausea, 96, 103
Neo Synephrine, 106
nerve damage, 91–94, 101–2
neurological checks. *See* monitoring

neurological status, 29–34
   emergency treatment, 107–8
   monitoring, 47–52, 54, 90–91, 101–3, 106
   post-operative, 62–63
neurosurgeons, 67–68
Newcastle endarterectomy trial, 11
non-valvular atrial fibrillation, 21
North American Symptomatic Carotid Endarterectomy Trial (NASCET), 12–13
numbness, 33

O

obstructions. *See* clots; emboli; thrombosis
occlusion catheters, 52, 54–56, 62, 83–87
ophthalmic artery, 31
ophthalmologic evaluation, 31–32
osteoporosis screening, 39

P

patch grafts, 58, 62, 87–89, 99
patient care, post-operative, 58
patient position during surgery, 52, 104–6
peripheral arterial screening, 39
phenylephrine (Neo Synephrine), 106
physicians' role in screenings, 117–18
plaque, 55–62, 64–65*figs*, 85–87
   dissectors, 58–61
   incision length, 83
   Pruitt-Inahara Shunt, 84*fig*
   ulcers, 13, 18, 20, 29–30, 45
pneumonia, 96
position, 52, 104–6
preoperative testing, 96–97
prevention, 3–4, 29–43, 109
   See also screening tests

prior strokes, 13, 20
Prolene sutures, 57
protamine, 54, 106
prothrombin time (PT), 25–26
Pruitt-Inahara Shunt, 79*fig*, 84*fig*
PTFE patch grafts, 88
pulmonary function tests, 96–97

Q

quality standards, 121
questions for surgeons, 67–100

R

racial differences, 37
radioactive Xenon, 70–72
recovery room, 90
recurrent laryngeal nerve, 53, 93–94, 101–2
re-endarterectomy, 98–99
renal artery stenosis, 43
research, 4–5, 10–14, 39–40, 112, 116
    double-blind studies, xviii
respiratory status, 90
retinal emboli, 32
rheumatic heart disease, 26
right angle clamps, 61
right angle dissectors, 59*fig*, 60
risks
   diabetes mellitus, 99
   surgery, 61–62, 91–98, 103
   morbidity and mortality, 11–12, 15, 48, 49
   re-endarterectomy, 99
   recurrence, 98–99
   stroke, 13–14, 19–20, 95, 112
Rob, C.G., xvii, 10
routine medical examinations, 109

S

saphenous vein grafts, 88
scalene blocks, 104–5
scarring, 91, 98–99
scheduling surgery, 96
screening tests, 4–5, 7, 35–40, 109, 110
   accuracy, 118
   atrial fibrillation, 5–6, 40
   auricular fibrillation, 7
   brain hemorrhage, 6
   cost-benefit analysis, 121–22
   costs, 26, 117, 121–22
   hypertension, 7, 40–41
   Life Line, 111–22
   National Stroke Association, 114
   physicians' role, 117–18
   quality standards, 121
   ultrasound, 110–21
sedation, 52, 69, 72, 102–6
seizures, 90
Sherman, D.G., 11
shortness of breath, 22
shunting, 51–52, 57, 62, 69, 71, 101–3
   procedures, 73–76, 84*fig*
shunts, 69–70, 77–82*figs*
   balloons, 79–84
   end points, 83–86
   natural thyroid, 53*fig*, 57*fig*
   side ports, 76–82
smoking, 13, 20, 97, 99, 109
Society of Vascular Technology, 39–40
sodium-heparin, 54
speech changes, 19, 33, 64–65*figs*
spring bulldog clamp, 54, 56

statistics, 1, 36
   atrial fibrillation, 26
   research trials, 12–14
   risks of stroke, 95, 108
   See also morbidity and mortality
straight dissector, 59*fig*
stroke, 1*def,* 75–76, 94–95
   risks, 72–73, 98, 101–3
   side ports, 79
   statistics, 95, 108
stump flow, 55
stump pressure, 70–71, 102
Sundt, Thoralf, xvii
Sundt Shunt, 77*fig*
superior laryngeal nerve, 53, 93–94
superior thyroid artery, 53–54, 62
surgeons, 15, 67–100
   morbidity and mortality, 48, 49*fig*
   qualifications, 45–46
surgery for carotid stenosis, 45–65
   checklist, 54, 61–62
   complications, 101–2
   indications, 45
   vs. medical management, 3, 36, 48
   monitoring, 101–2
   patient position on the table, 104–6
   procedures, 52–65
   risks, 62–63, 91–99, 103
   suturing, 52–53, 57, 61, 83, 89
   team, 95
   See also shunting
suturing, 52–53, 57, 61, 83, 89
symptoms of carotid stenosis, 29–34
syncope, 34

T

INDEX

Teflon injections, 93–94
Teflon patch grafts, 88
Textbook of Medicine, 9th Edition (Cecil & Loeb), 7
Thompson, Jessie, xvii
thoracic surgeons, 67–68
thrombosis, 7–10, 43, 90, 108
    atrial fibrillation, 42
    carotid endarterectomy, 101–2
    post-operative, 58, 62
    timing of surgery, 95–96
TIAs. *See* transient ischemic attacks
timing of surgery, 95–96
tissue plasminogen activator (t-PA), 107–8
tongue weakness and coordination, 92
t-PA. *See* tissue plasminogen activator
transcranial Doppler, 70–72, 102
transient ischemic attacks (TIAs), 10–13, 18*fig,* 19*def,* 20, 65*fig,* 90–91
    diagnosis, 29–34
    emergency treatment, 107–8
    timing of surgery, 95–96

U

ulcerated plaque, 13, 20, 29–30, 18*fig,* 45, 64–65*figs*
    See also plaque
ultrasound, 4–5, 32, 42, 47, 57
    accuracy, 118
    echocardiograms, 23
    Life Line Screenings, 111–22
    screening tests, 35–40, 109–22

V

vagus nerve, 53, 93–94
valvular atrial fibrillation, 21
vascular surgeons, 67–68

VA Symptomatic Carotid Endarterectomy Trial, 14
ventricular aneurysms, 26
Versed, 52, 102, 104–6
vertebral arteries, 16*fig*, 17, 34
   stenosis, 10–11
   tests, 42
   ultrasound, 47
vessel loops, 52, 61
vision changes, 19, 30–31, 64*fig.*
voice changes, 93–94

W
Walker, A.E., 9
warfarin, 23, 25, 43
weakness, 33
World Health Organization, 25

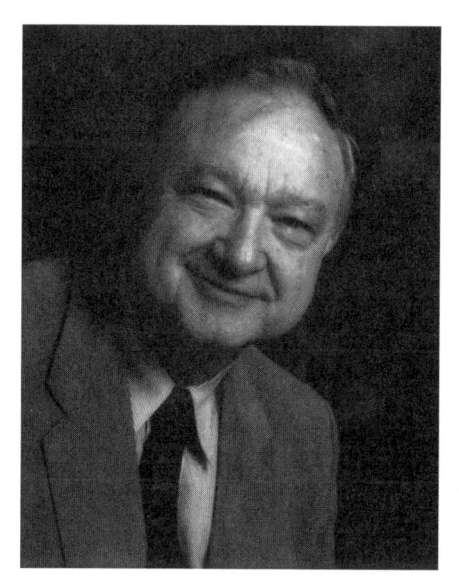

About the Author

J. Crayton Pruitt, M.D., F.A.C.S., was born in Jefferson, South Carolina, and is a graduate of Emory University and the Emory University School of Medicine in Atlanta, Georgia. He completed his internship at Mound Park Hospital in St. Petersburg and his residency at Bowman Gray School of Medicine and the North Carolina Baptist Hospital.

Dr. Pruitt began his private practice of thoracic, general, and cardiovascular surgery in St. Petersburg, Florida, in 1963. He is certified by the American Board of Surgery and the American Board of Thoracic Surgery. He is co-developer of the Pruitt-Inahara Carotid Shunt.

He is thought to have performed more carotid endarterectomies than any surgeon in the world. His research for the National Cancer Institute resulted in a Certificate of Merit Award from the American Medical Association's Section of Preventive Medicine. He has published numerous scientific papers, has been a Clinical Assistant Professor at the University of South Florida School of Medicine, and is Director of the Vascular Institute of Florida.

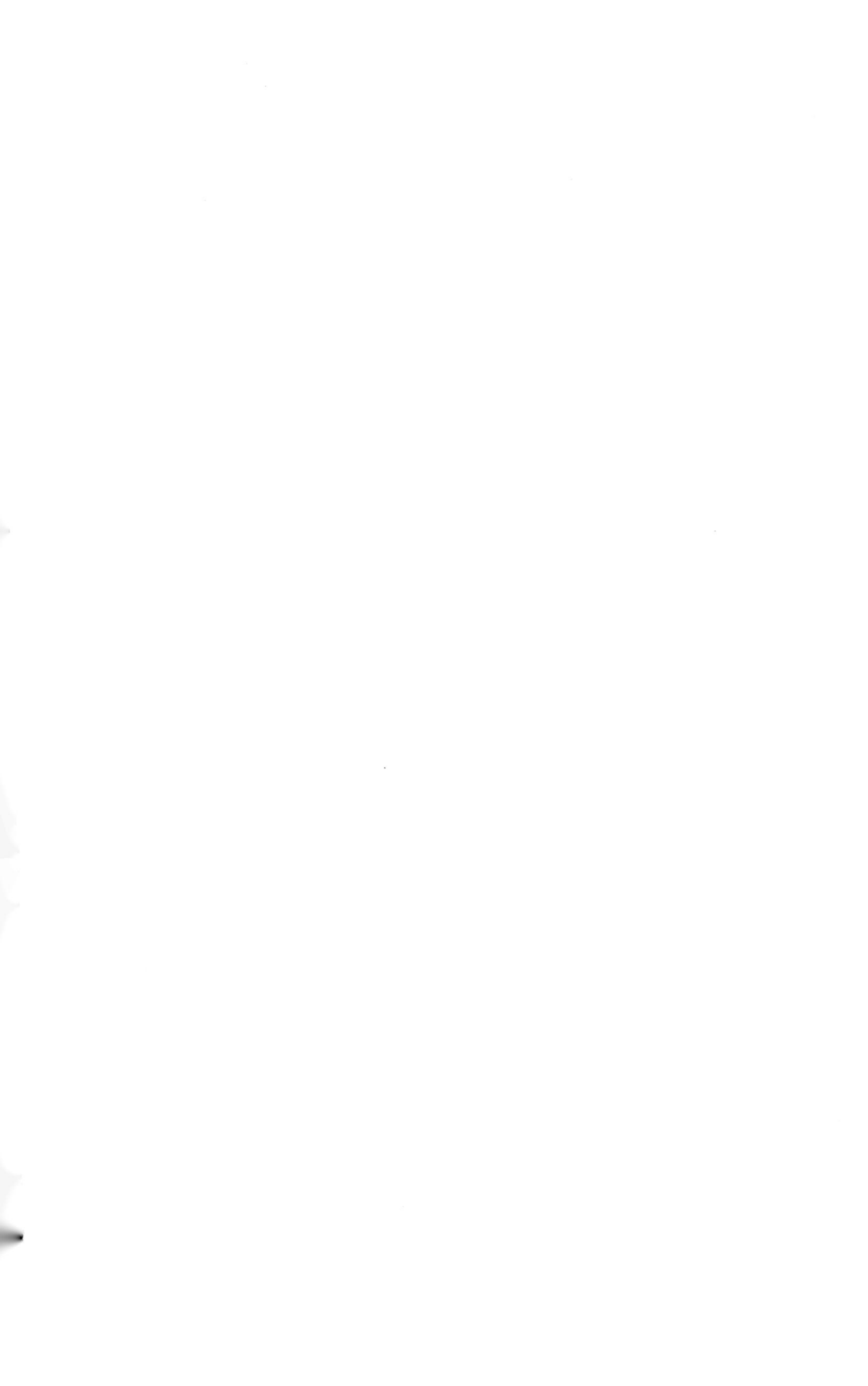